"Every so often a book comes along that catches you off guard. It has something special - even wonderful - in it and yet you don't exactly know what it is. As I read *Your Script for Hope*, I felt as if I was being brought along a journey into my own heart, into the author's heart, and into all our collective hearts."

   – **Allan Doane**, Computer Scientist and Board Certified Hypnotist, Ojai, CA, USA

"*Your Script for Hope* is perfect for all of us on our journey through the Human Condition. Whether battling an illness, healing from past trauma, or just the journey of life. This book encompasses tools and suggestions to live your best life filled with joy, experience, and LOVE."

   – **Jeanne Klein**, Business Owner, Reading, PA, USA

"Author Petra Frese is truly an angel. It takes a special soul and a servant's heart to help bring balance and peace to ones' body, mind, spirit, and soul."

   – **Michael Bizzoso**, Manager, Macungie, PA, USA

"*Your Script for Hope* breaks all the rules when talking about death and dying. Death is scary. Death is feared. And why? Petra takes you on a real-life journey with one of her clients where she removes that fear and gracefully replaces it with love and peace."

   – **Donna Reynolds**, Business Owner, Phillipsburg, NJ, USA

"In *Your Script for Hope*, you have a guide; an angel on earth to help you through troubling and trying times. Share this book with everyone you know for no matter what their situation - there is hope."

— **Doug Norman**, Marine Corps Veteran,
Easton, PA, USA

"A warmly written, easy to read, straight to the point book, that on top of it reveals the mystic side behind a devastating diagnosis as well. It provides a precise overview on what happens and how you can cope with and manage it best."

— **Marco Muraro**, Intuitive Mental-Life Coach,
Zürich, ZH, Switzerland

"This is a heartfelt book, where Petra speaks her truth with honesty, compassion, insight, clarity, and most importantly, with love and hopefulness. It provides simple explanations and practical advice for application in the reader's life. I hope it will continually find its way into the hands of those who can learn and grow from its lessons."

— **Leslie Adam**, Instructor, Wexford, PA, USA

"Encouraging, enlightening, and empowering. Amazing Read!"

— **Scott Saylor**, Sales Specialist,
Saucon Valley, PA, USA

"*Your Script for Hope* provides a patter and an action plan for the empowering journey of discovering the light at the end of a tunnel. This book is a warm introduction to the gifts that Petra imbues upon each and every one of her clients and students. May we all find a bit more hope in reading her words."

— **Caitlin Allison**, Clinical Social Worker and Hypnotherapist, Charlotte, NC, USA

"This book isn't just for those dealing with a frightening diagnosis, it's also for the caretakers. It's for those who need a guide who's been there, that they can trust to nudge them back to love. This book is really for anyone who has ever wondered whether or not they have the power to heal themselves or anyone else."

— **Robin Bennett**, Writer and Marketing Strategist, Atlanta, GA, USA

"This book is long-overdue. Finally, a wonderful book that teaches us how to be whole and present in this experience."

— **Joe Crisanti**, Hypnotist, Flemington, NJ, USA

"Mrs. Frese has provided an all-encompassing guide to enable one to live through these situations, and has benevolently shared engaging personal experiences to enable us to learn through empathy where direct experiences would not avail us."

— **Emeka Okoo Uka**, Lawyer and Entrepreneur, Abuja, Nigeria

"This book is full of compassion, love, and powerful tools. Learn with Frese how to keep your ability to act in a self-determined way. I'm keeping this book like a treasure."

– **Bettina Kübler**, Programmer,
Oberarth, SZ, Switzerland

"I absolutely love this book. It touches on so many of life's feelings, emotions, thoughts, obstacles and so much more which we all experience at one time or another in life. I do highly recommend this book to anyone!

– **Debbie Eschbach**, Business Owner,
Northampton, PA, USA

"Frese's warm and precise storytelling makes it an easy read. *Your Script for Hope* creates hope when realizing that our souls are always connected whatever transition phase we are in - the author actually proves it to you."

– **Murièle Solange Bolay**, Empathetic
Strategist, Zug, ZG, Switzerland

Your Script for Hope

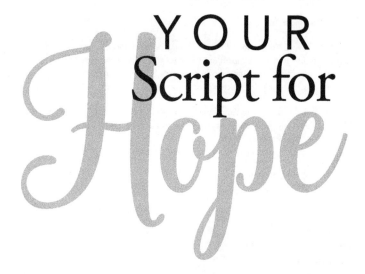

YOUR
Script for
Hope

Overcome a
Devastating Diagnosis

DR. H.C. PETRA FRESE

NEW YORK

LONDON • NASHVILLE • MELBOURNE • VANCOUVER

Your Script for Hope

Overcome a Devastating Diagnosis

Published in New York, New York, by Morgan James Publishing in partnership with Difference Press. Morgan James is a trademark of Morgan James, LLC. www.MorganJamesPublishing.com

ISBN 9781642796278 paperback
ISBN 9781642796285 eBook
ISBN 9781642796292 audio
Library of Congress Control Number: 2019942345

Cover Design by:
Megan Dillon
megan@creativeninjadesigns.com

Interior Design by:
Chris Treccani
www.3dogcreative.net

Author Photo by:
Judy Reinford

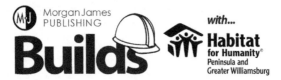

Morgan James is a proud partner of Habitat for Humanity Peninsula and Greater Williamsburg. Partners in building since 2006.

Get involved today! Visit
MorganJamesPublishing.com/giving-back

For Stella.

TABLE OF CONTENTS

FOREWORD

Petra Frese's life began on a fairly isolated place on earth, the GDR (German Democratic Republic), a country that does not exist any longer, but this fact has not kept her from dreaming big.

The first time I met Petra was in Switzerland in May 2013 in a hypnosis and hypnotherapy class that I taught. She stood out then, and she stands out today. She became not only a remarkable hypnotherapist creating miracles almost daily but also an exemplary instructor who passes on this passion for the subject to her students.

Petra is a rare breed of person. Her roots are in science, but she has managed to see beyond biochemical formulas and statistics and see the soul that lives in all of us. She was a volunteer in the firefighter brigade in Switzerland, and you would never guess that this delicate and soft-spoken woman can fight like a lioness if it comes to braving some of the worst that life can throw at you. She shows you how you can get back the control over your life, even in the process of dying – but also understand how to fight right, stay focused, fight with a strategy, fight using your strongest tool you have available to you: Your subconscious mind! Petra is the right ally to have at your side if you have received a devastating diagnosis. She brings light in the form of hope and love to places where there can be a lot of dark and fear and pain.

She has brought all her valuable real-life experience and the beautiful inner wisdom gained by it, to paper. She shares with us these remarkable insights, into what so many of us one day may face unexpectedly, but one never really can prepare for, despite knowing that this is also part of life.

Petra defied the odds and she fought hard to create the life she now has – helping, guiding, soothing, teaching others about life – and death – and how to fight as hard, focused, and yet eloquent for life as possible, but to also fight hard to transition with ease, dignity, and in peace, embracing love, being able to let go, and change over smoothly. She can help you find peace within, to forgive others and especially yourself, and let go of all things past that hurt or scarred and embrace with a clear mind the challenges that may lie ahead.

Your Script for Hope is as much a book about life as it is about death. It is about hope for life, and the love for the life one eventually leaves behind, ultimately accepting the next step on your terms. This book will guide and teach the affected not by some theoretical approach, but by real-life example, as Petra had, herself, a life full of life-threatening challenges that she had to overcome. Her life is a mirror and inspiration at the same time. Her being alive today, as well as her daughter, are the living proof of that.

"What the mind can conceive, the body can achieve" is not just a catchy phrase, but Petra will show you step-by-step how to work on turning the odds in your favor again, but also how to go about letting go.

Get back in control. Get in charge of your healing or, if need be, your transitioning – but get back in charge, take command, as you will not be guided by fear, despair, or pain any longer, but with love.

Let Petra be your guide and inspiration in showing you how. It's a good decision – it may be the only hope there is. I know I would.

– Hansruedi Wipf

FOREWORD

If you are keen to learn from Petra or to hear about our very personal story, please skip this. If you want to hear about a different perspective of the same story, stay on!

This is based on philosophy and science. The resulting tension developing between Petra's and my view on the world or *Weltanschauung* is so powerful she thought that this divergent aspect might help you to get a better grasp on the topic.

I am writing these lines 36'000 feet above ground. Trying to be closer to heaven, the angels and God. This is a business trip to Miami. Petra doesn't need to travel in an airplane to be closer to Spirit. She knows, is aware, sensitive enough to allow her to travel with her mind and at the same time to stay on the ground. I adore her for this capacity.

In the process of Petra writing the book, we had many arguments. We represent opposites, me being the analytical scientist – skepticism is the scientist's nature. Petra, herself, is a scientist as well but grew into being spiritual for reasons explained later in the book. Even if you are into astrology you will find out that her being Libra, me being an Aries, we are on opposite sides of the zodiac cycle. Very different and yet complementing each other, more than 25 years by now. Astrology was not for me, as I could not explain it. Petra brought this knowledge closer to home. I learned that there is something to it, which I cannot explain or understand but experience nonetheless.

Petra went from pure and applied science to a holistic view utilizing hypnosis, shamanism, and other transcendental states to heal. Our opposite views led to many controversies and even fights at home with fruitful outcomes. To get there, we rooted for each other passionately to search, understand, develop, and apply the holistic concept on our distinct philosophies to further grow and improve together.

You, dear reader, can rest assured. We fought these battles for you. She was once my Ph.D. student, and she developed and grew into being my partner, wife, mom of our daughter – and always believing in us.

What you will read below is the essence and synthesis of two very different perspectives. Coined by experiences lived through together. Interpreted and assimilated differently, based on culture, upbringing, and mindset.

These discussions, often late at night after work, were very exhausting, and made me desperate to find common ground. Often, we did not achieve this right away, although eventually we did, which in turn allowed our partnership to grow even deeper and making it more fulfilling than ever.

What did I learn from Petra? Body. Mind. Spirit. Soul. These four elements engrained in the Native American culture and other philosophies or religions to varying degrees are everywhere, and must stay in balance to be healthy, successful, happy, and loving. In the end it boils down to LOVE.

In my opinion the power of the mind is underrated, the influence is not even properly studied yet. In her book, Petra describes the positive effects of the mindset on serious illnesses, for example, cancer. The general assumption is that cancer is a result of a genetic disorder. The cell machinery wreaking havoc can either be inherited or happen as a result of mutations acquired by environment, lifestyle, or just by chance. Therefore, the generally accepted cure for this terrible disease is surgery, chemotherapy, and radiation. Target it, remove it and kill it. The appalling side-effects on the body and mind are usually not discussed for various reasons. Is this really the way to go? Is it that simple?

I was under the same impression but, inspired by my wife, my view has changed. I applied the new viewpoint on what I had learned before: How in our DNA, the genes express themselves via a process called transcription into RNA and then via translation into proteins, suddenly realizing how complex and astounding these processes really are. The enormous magnitude of influences from timing, hormones, toxins, vitamins, further mutations,

RNA-DNA interactions and protein DNA interactions, epigenetics and many more allow for healthy or sick cells to develop, growth of cancer, or remission.

Let me illustrate the complexity with a simple analogy: In case you play the guitar, you know that there are generally six strings. Each tuned to a specific note: EADGBE.

The wonderful music you will hear is the result of what? The guitar, the body so to speak? The EADGBE strings, the DNA made from four nucleotides called GATC? The fingers, the mind or the RNA, peptides, and proteins? Or the emotions of the musician, the mood, the soul which result in Pop, Rock, Soul, Jazz, Hip-hop and many other music genres? Or even Spirit? I believe it is all of the above!

You see where I am getting at. If that is true, then the influence of the mind, spirit, and soul on our body and thus illnesses as even cancer cannot be neglected. The influence of these elements is very powerful especially when coupled with conventional medicine to produce miraculous results as Petra will highlight in the following compelling chapters which are filled with amazing case studies and recipes for hope.

For me personally, this holistic approach filled with love also changed my professional career significantly. I am an experienced manager leading teams globally and very successfully, driven, I might say, to provide leadership with heart.

For you, Petra's book will demonstrate that regardless of how tragic the situation seems to be, as our traditional, reasoned thinking, that we were conditioned to follow makes us believe, there is always hope. Hope because of the inexplicable, the spiritual forces, and the power they have in the form and shape of our mind which this is creating. Our mind, in turn, then influences the cellular functions leading to recovery or allowing us to find peace with the transition to follow. Either way, it is a miracle.

– Dr. Dirk Frese

INTRODUCTION

"Pure logic is the ruin of the Spirit."
– Antoine de Saint-Exupéry

Stella is sitting in the dark. She got here a while ago. Since she has received her devastating diagnosis, the dark has an even deeper meaning for her.

She uses her time to think. She wonders about the meaning of life and other philosophical and spiritual questions. What is the deeper meaning of life? Life is a journey, a ride with surprises. Nobody prepares us for this kind of adventure at school. We need to learn and understand life in our own way and at our own pace. Life is about learning. But what is death about? Nobody teaches us what death is about and how to die. What is it to die? Why do we fear death? Does dying always have to go hand in hand with pain and exhaustion and fear and worries and grief? Does it always have to be a roller coaster of emotions? Why is death a taboo topic? Why is it taboo and yet it happens to all of us?

Stella is very familiar with the roller coaster of emotions. She worries a lot. She worries about her family. How will they manage life once she will be gone? She wants to live with her family as the caring mom and the loving wife she is and always wanted to be. She does not want to disappoint her loved ones!

How can she handle the stress and the pain? She doesn't want her kids to see her suffer. She doesn't want her husband to feel helpless. She doesn't want her cat to not get fed on time.

Stella needs to find a way to sleep again at night. She wants to find a way to rest, to recharge. She needs to find help, support, compassion, and an outlet for her mammoth amount of anger. She desperately needs someone who will guide her to master this unbearable challenge in her life. In the time she has left, she wants to enjoy life to the fullest. She wants to gratefully embrace the quality moments and the sparks of light for herself and for her family. She wants to see the light again and not be captured by despair and fear of the unknown. She wants to live with love and to die in love.

She needs a miracle. *Now!*

I will take you, my dear reader, on a journey following an apparently unalterable diagnosis, a seemingly irrevocable situation. I will share with you case studies from my practices in Switzerland and the United States of America. The names of my clients have been changed. However, circumstances, treatments, procedures, and outcomes are purest, simplest truth. Any similarity to people you know might be sheer coincidence. I will explain the course of action step by step and fill it with examples and practical exercises that are easy to apply. By the end of your reading, you will have received a guidebook with clear action steps, the reasoning behind them, and why this could help you or the people you care for. By the end of the book, I hope you feel understood, encouraged, and filled with hope.

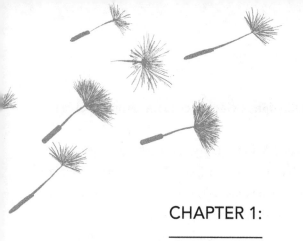

CHAPTER 1:

Reaching for the Stars

"No problem can be solved from the same level of consciousness that created it."

– Albert Einstein

It has been a long day for me. My last client had left more than an hour ago. I took the time to finish my paperwork and to review the day. Now I'm ready to go home. I switch off the lights, leave my office, and lock the door. It is already dark outside, and I had forgotten to switch on the lights in the client waiting area. Nobody had complained. I'm hanging on to my thoughts, and while turning the key, I feel a presence. I turn around, and there she is. A shadow, just slightly visible thanks to the streetlight next to the window. I startle! I'm shaking. I'm frightened. I'm rushing to find the light switch to ease the situation at least a little bit.

"Who are you? What are you doing here?" My voice sounds louder than I expected it to. She does not move at all. Very softly she answers, "I am Stella." Silence. I'm able to turn on the light, and now I can see her. She has beautiful eyes. She's very slender, sitting sunken down, weak, no body tension. She is wearing a turban.

My mind is working on turbo-speed: Was another client scheduled? Had I missed an appointment? Had I known anything about her? What am I missing? Why don't I have any information from my assistant? What was going on here?

I find myself standing in front of her and I hear myself asking, "What can I do for you?"

Stella's voice is very mild, almost a whisper. "I need an appointment."

"Certainly, I can give you an appointment. My next available time slot is in two months." Politely, I add, "It would have been okay to just call, and my assistant would have given you an appointment. You would not have to sit in the dark and wait for me."

A teeny-weeny smile flits over her face.

"I have called, and I know that the next appointment is available in two months." Pause. "I don't have two months." Pause. "My medical doctors told me that I have two maybe three more weeks to live."

It's almost midnight. It doesn't take many words to make me reopen the office. We team up.

As professionally as possible, she provides me with all the data, with all the facts and information I need to know so that we can efficiently start to work together.

She has lung cancer, stage four. She went through all possible treatments, modern Western medicine, the whole nine yards, and a lot of methods of alternative medicine. The prognosis is unacceptable for her.

Stella, in her mid-fifties, is a mom - mommy with all her heart. She and her husband have a wonderful daughter and a wonderful son together. She loves them dearly. I learn that her husband is a lot older than she is. They have prepared themselves according to the life-expectancy statistics. It was not part of the plan that she would leave this earthly lifetime before him. She is gushing. Her voice is becoming stronger and stronger with each sentence she says. She is extremely short on breath. We talk intensely about her worries, her concerns, and her beliefs, dreams, and wishes.

We both believe in reincarnation. We both find out that we have not been raised with this belief. We have the right to make a decision to believe in something based on information, based on our thoughts, on our feelings, and on our experiences. We also have the right to change our beliefs if we understand that something else makes more sense to us now, maybe based on new experiences or new information.

She worries about her family. She wants to see her children get married. She is motherly proud of her kids. They are good at school and active in sports. They study diligently and have fun and fool around like healthy teenagers. Her husband is very loving and hard-working. He spends too many hours in their family-owned business. Yes, she knows, he does it for his family. She knows that this is his way of showing his love. More and more often, she misses his presence. She misses talking with him; she misses talking also about her cancer illness. She is aware of her demands and that it is impossible to fulfill her desires. She is aware of how much she puts onto him. She is aware that it takes a superhuman-effort to handle her in this situation sometimes. She is not a bad person. She just doesn't know better. She is desperate.

She is extremely stressed. It's almost impossible for her to rest. She doesn't know how to recharge and how to get this noisy chitchat in her head to stop, at least for a while. Sleep has become a foreign word to her. Good quality sleep seems to have been too long ago to even be remembered.

Her knowledge about food and healthy eating is vast. She cooks for her family whenever possible, but still it is virtually impossible for Stella to eat properly. In contrast, it is very easy for Stella to feed their cat with healthy, delicious food on time. She can make her cat happy but not her beloved family anymore. That is her biggest problem. This is what makes her feel so guilty, so ashamed, so unworthy. She loves her family. She needs her family to be happy. Her family is her reason to live. Her reason to live is love.

Besides chemotherapy and radiation treatment, she has tried acupuncture, kinesiology, homeopathy, reiki, herbology, and many other modalities. What else could she do? Self-doubt, hopelessness, and fear have taken over. She doesn't know how to cope with her anxieties and her emotional and physical pain.

She needs help. She needs someone who knows more about this journey. She needs someone who can guide her. She needs someone who travels with her. She needs her miracle! Now!

What is a miracle for you? What does miracle mean to you?

I ask Stella this question, and she slams with her flat hand on the table, the glass tabletop clanks: "One year! I need one year!" We both grow stiff for a moment. We both have different reasons for our pause. Stella is astonished about her boldness. My analytical mind immediately questions the restriction. Why one year? Why only one year? My conscious mind contemplates this one, single year. She is still young, she has adolescent children. Why only one year? I know what can be achieved from my own experiences. I also know that each and every one of us knows exactly what we need. We talk about it, and Stella realizes that this is her deepest inner wish. She subconsciously knew what she needed, and somehow it just had erupted out of her. Being very vulnerable and honest, she also discloses that she is constantly told to fight.

Fighting is not what she wants; it is against her nature. She would rather ride it out her way. By the end of her lifetime, she wants to have understood the important lessons of life. She does not want to have any business unfinished. She wants to be at peace with herself and her loved ones. In her last chapter of life, she wants to be safe and happy and also loved. Stella wants to die in peace and with love. That is the miracle she is longing for.

Over the course of fifteen months, we created Stella's miracle. Her MDs couldn't explain it. They didn't find a way to understand or rationalize this unexpected life prolongation, much longer than the predicted two to three weeks and paired with such a high quality of life. Two and a half weeks short of one year after we had met for the very first time, Stella informed me on the phone, "It is starting now." We both knew that she was right, and we shifted gears. She has had a close to normal life for eleven months and two weeks. She lived very consciously, went to work part-time, was pain-free most of the time, respected her lowered levels of energy, and enjoyed all the gifts of life, all the happy moments to the fullest. Stella had finished all her open businesses and had gotten her affairs in order. We embarked on Stella's last leg of her earthly journey together. The logical mind is not capable of grasping this. Her doctors are all of the same opinion, that it is a miracle. As a priceless side-effect, we, Stella and I, developed a very deep connection and close friendship. Our link is unconditional love.

Why do you think I can help you create your own unique miracle? What do you know about me? Why me?

Stella says she had tried everything. Every method was used in an isolated way. Every method she had applied gave a little help but not what she had wished for. She had not worked with her higher mind yet. And nobody had seen the big picture. Nobody had connected the dots. Stella whispers: "You are my last hope." That's why she is here, in my office, no matter what time it is, midnight doesn't matter. What matters are the two or three weeks she has left. That is what matters - because of her family, because love matters.

Together, we design a plan specifically for Stella. This plan adjusts to her unique circumstances, to her unique situation. It consists of managing stress, mastering pain, recharging during sleep, incorporating healthy eating, activating self-healing powers, controlling fears, bringing her affairs in order and much, much more. We break the plan down into doable steps. I give Stella the tools and teach her how to use them, which enables her to put the plan into practice. A plan is worth diddly-squat until it is implemented, until it is put into action. I hold space for her, and I keep her accountable. Whenever she struggles, I help her through the challenge. Together we travel far, so much farther than she could have traveled alone. I am her cheerleader, her support, her backup, her protection, her companion, her lighthouse, her tour guide. How can I be all this? How do I know the way? I have been there. I have traveled this route, more than once… I made it back. I am familiar with the journey called dying.

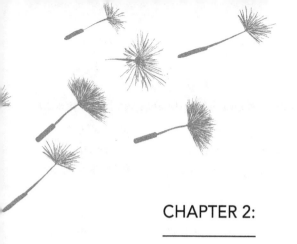

CHAPTER 2:

Little Did They Know

"There are only two ways to live your life.
One is as though nothing is a miracle. The other
is as though everything is a miracle."
– Albert Einstein

Little did I know as I was playing with the angels as a little girl that nobody else in my family could see, hear, or feel them like I did. To me, this was normal. I had no understanding that for many other people, including my parents a different normal existed.

I grew up in a little village in the German Democratic Republic as an only child in a pretty ordinary family. I was sick a lot. I will not dive into the details of the learning curve of my super sensitive soul during my childhood. I will just give you an overview. I had fun at school, and

I was a dreamer. I dreamed big dreams, and still do. At the age of nine, I proclaimed to my parents that I would grow up and then go to America. My parents laughed out loud about this absurd, and at that impossible idea of my childish mind.

I finished school, went on to vocational school and later graduated from Humboldt University in Berlin with a Master of Science engineering degree. Additionally, I studied molecular genetics and medicine for a couple of semesters. I experienced the reunification of Germany firsthand, living in East-Berlin during that time. My doctoral research studies brought me to the Technical University in West-Berlin, where I studied the science of aging. There I met my husband who had just graduated with his doctorate in biochemistry, and I pursued our research. He was dictated by his boss to become my supervisor. At first, we didn't get along very well but he took his mentoring very seriously and, as he says, he found his diamond in the rough. We are happily married and have a wonderful daughter together.

Even though life polishes me, sometimes I'm still very rough.

Besides the cultural differences between East- and West-Germany that we had to overcome, we had to face multiple, severe health-threatening situations very early in our young, fragile relationship. We found out about my pregnancy on a Wednesday and the following Saturday, I ended up in the ER of the Charité, one of the leading hospitals in the world. Little did I know that I would rarely leave the hospital for the next thirty-two weeks.

I want to give you hope! I want to encourage you. I want to show you what miracles are possible. I want you to trust - to trust the power of your inner mind. I want you to trust yourself! I want you to make your decision. Decide for your journey, decide for your miracle. Choose love! This is my reason why I am sharing these very personal experiences with you.

We had to make a decision, right then. We would either let this unscheduled pregnancy naturally cease, or we would move heaven and earth and fight for this little, unborn being growing inside of my body. We had not been prepared for that at all. Our plans didn't include commitment yet. They didn't include long-term goals. We both trust in higher guidance, and with only one look into each other's eyes, all doubt was surrendered.

Having two children in Heaven, carrying the loss of two children in my treasure chest of life experiences, I was rather uncomfortable to deal with. I did not trust. I didn't trust any medical professional. They had not been able – in my young, grieving mind I actually questioned their willingness – to keep my babies safe. All the trauma, all that grieving pain was reawakening suddenly. I did not trust life. I did not trust myself. I did not trust anything or anyone. Maybe I trusted the father of my unborn baby. His father was an OB-GYN, who was calm, warm-hearted, down to earth, well-versed, and I felt his loving personality from the very first minute we met. We had an extremely special bond. I talked myself into at least trying to trust him as, at the very least, I knew he would want to do right by his son and his grandchild.

There was a truly rare abnormality with my blood. Since close to no research and almost no knowledge was available about this blood condition, it was put into the category of autoimmune disease. The MDs tried to figure out a treatment plan for me. Based on the little information available, they handled it as trial and error. On top of this, I had bleedings and preterm contractions and spent 24/7 in a hospital bed, infusion in both arms. I wasn't allowed to get up and use the bathroom or shower. I was constantly throwing up and dramatically losing weight. My mind had more than enough time to spiral down into the realms of fear, concerns, and imagery of the worst outcome. It required all my vigor to guide my mind to safe places over and over again, to happy moments, to good images and to the delightful search of our baby's name.

In the middle of the sixth month of pregnancy, my squadron of medical professionals gathered around my bed. I had recently started to like the head physician of the intensive care unit. My due date was on his birthday. A little trust had been established. My husband-to-be was standing next to me on my right side, my chief physician took position at the foot end of the bed, and all the other white-coats gathered around. They filled up the room while I was lying in the bed with my body inclined up the legs to weaken the premature contractions and with an IV in each arm. Now the meeting could start. The big cheese, seemingly unaffected, started his statement only looking at my baby's father. "Dr. Frese, I have to inform you that your baby is almost dead, and your wife is not far away from dying, either. There is nothing else we can do."

Shock.

Silence.

They wanted him to immediately decide to abort my pregnancy to at least have a tiny bit of a chance to save my life.

Silence again.

My head was spinning. I could not grasp a single thought, let alone think it through. Lightning flashed through my head. Merry-go-round. Roller coaster. Thoughts. Emotions. Fear. Wrath. Why don't they talk to me?! Why don't they ask *me*?! Why don't they even look at me?! Am I still alive? I checked my breath and realized, I had stopped breathing. "Okay" I internally said to myself. "Breathe! Let's see whether you can breathe. This would mean you are alive." I continued breathing. Whilst I was occupied with my breathing, my future husband made a decision. What the MDs had offered to him was not an option for us!

He demanded a meeting with the medical staff. He would come up with a treatment plan for me. He would take over complete liability. Yes, he would sign all the release documents. This was not a request; this was an order!

He saved my life. He saved our daughter's life. Ever since, I have trusted this man boundlessly. His father was all in. The anger this meeting had kindled in me became a wildfire. I became a force. I heroically fought my daily inner combat, not against someone or something. I fought *for* something. I fought *for* our baby. My driving force was love.

As a consequence of my high-risk pregnancy, the decision was made very early on that I would deliver through a C-section. Month seven of my pregnancy went by pretty smoothly, so my head physician felt confident enough to change his mind and announced it to be a natural birth. We imperatively wanted to legalize our relationship, especially since my prospects of surviving this labor were minimal. My MDs strongly encouraged us to get my affairs in order. I had already done this. Secretly, I had prepared for my suicide. In the improbable case I should survive and my baby did not, I was prepared. Everything was planned through and artfully organized in secrecy. The physicians obviously didn't expect this child to be alive after delivery and they did not have much hope for me either. From a scientific standpoint, it seemed to be impossible to endure those amounts of high doses of various medical drugs over such a long time. If at all alive, this baby would not be healthy. Dirk, the baby's father, and I were tirelessly battling for our wishes and dreams.

After week thirty-six, I got permission to get up from my hospital bed. We took the chance and got married. It was wonderfully amusing for our families. We had a nice, small wedding. Forty-two hours later, our daughter was born naturally after only five and a half hours of labor. She did not cry. No visible vital signs. The whole medical staff took her away. I was left behind, alone. I wanted to scream, but no tone came out of me. None. Not a single one. After an eternity, a nurse came back to me and took my hand. "She is alive."

Fairly exhausted, they slowly came back and wanted to finish up with me. After a while, my precious baby was brought into my room and I could see her. I was completely overwhelmed. I was not neither able nor allowed to touch or hold her. She was taken care of by medical professionals, and so was I. I was losing blood, more than my body could handle. My husband was the one who realized that I was bleeding like I was in a slaughterhouse. He alerted the doctors who, at that time, seemed to believe that the baby and I were fine after we survived delivery. But it was not over yet. An old scar from a previous delivery had burst. I suffered a uterus rupture. I needed emergency surgery. As fast as they could, they provided the best medical help. I felt comfortably indifferent. I gradually drifted away in slow-motion.

The next thing I remember was observing the scene from a couple of feet above. The nurses and doctors were hectically working on something. Oh, that's my body.

Amused, I thought about busy ants. Weightless and free of any discomfort, I levitated. My gateway was a short black tunnel leading into an indescribable, brilliant, bright, warm light. I reached the light and it felt phenomenal. Figure-like shapes awaited me. I could distinguish their faces. I recognized some of them. I was happy to meet with all of them. I felt safe, welcomed, at home. Abruptly, I was stopped. "What?!? Why are you blocking my way?" I felt myself thinking. She answered in a mellow yet certain voice, "You are here to learn, to grow. We allow you to catch a glimpse. Your time has not come yet. Your mission is not done yet. You need to go back. They need you."

"But… but… but…" I pleaded to stay.

"We want you here. You are very welcomed here with us. We are waiting for you. It is not your time. You need to go back. You are needed over there."

"What do I need to do? What is so important?"

"We let you know." In that moment, I was all-knowing, omniscient. I felt complete.

The familiar voice with the flawless face was my great-aunt who I had met two or three times as a child before she had passed away many years ago – she left no wiggle room. I had to go back to Earth. I was pushed by an unthinkable energy. No way to hold on, no chance to not be kicked back.

Ughhhh, back into my body, back into weight and pain and fear. It felt like 30 seconds, maybe one minute. In earthly time, it was six hours and forty minutes later. I had been in heaven. My husband went through hell. He, holding our newborn baby-girl in his guarding arms, was told that the MDs had lost me. They had no clue what else they could do. I just didn't respond to anything. Helpless, hopeless, he was given the message that he would be a sole parent. It took me six years to talk with him about my excursion.

Fast forward. I'm skipping all the small, the medium, and the big events in my life. I only focus on some of the huge ones. Fast forward ten years. Vanessa, our beautiful daughter, is bright and second to none, remarkably curious, diligently studying, intelligently humorous, monstrously stubborn, exceptionally empathetic, and has a giant sense of fairness. She makes us thoroughly happy although she demands a lot of energy.

On June 6th, two days after she got her booster vaccination against tick-borne meningitis, at bedtime she found tons of excuses to not be quiet in her room and fall asleep. Late in the evening she called me again, which made me angry. She could not move her legs. First, I took it as just another excuse from her. I was quick to realize that it was no joke. She really could not move her legs. She did not feel her feet and legs. My anger instantly transformed into major concern. Alarmed, we immediately drove her to the next hospital with pediatricians. She was barely conscious as we arrived about thirty-five minutes later. Her condition declined continuously. The first doctor on duty in the medical unit kicked us out with the lackadaisical words "That child is just tired." He did not even bother to examine Vanessa.

I yelled, "I know my child! I have had her for ten years now! I know how she is when she is tired!" We had no other choice than to leave. We checked back into that hospital again instantaneously. Another doctor determined the situation on the spot and rushed her into the emergency unit and shortly after that, they sprinted to admit her to the intensive care unit. They did not have the slightest idea what she was suffering from. Many different tests, examinations, analyses - nothing gave a result that would have led to a diagnosis, which would have warranted a specific treatment. It was all a shot in the dark. Her condition became worse and worse. She was in horrible pain, needed morphine. Her cognitive abilities had vanished. The only people she still would recognize were her father and me. Mom and Dad were the only two words she could speak. All language, all colors, all senses had disappeared. She was completely paralyzed. Paralysis was encroaching on her respiratory center too. The giant number of medical examinations over eight weeks had given us the virtually useless insight. She was suffering from a deep-seated brain infection known as encephalitis. Nobody had a scientific explanation of where it came from nor any idea how to treat it. All academic knowledge culminated in two sentences: "She will not survive the night. You better say goodbye to her."

NOOOO!!!

We frantically vortexed in despair, close to literally losing our minds.

I stayed with her, exactly like I had for the last eight weeks. I prayed, I cursed, I begged, I cried, I bargained. I talked to her in love. In that very night, I entirely captured the true meaning of *unconditional* love.

The next morning, she was still breathing. Almost wordless, making myself unapologetically clear through body language, I signed all release documents, and we took her home. I became her first and sole caregiver. I constantly talked to her. I talked to her no matter whether she was conscious or not. I talked to her day and night and night and day. The phases when she was conscious became longer and longer. After some weeks, she did not fall unconscious anymore. We worked our butts off. We cried together, and we laughed together. Once again, we laughed together! I never stopped talking to her. I had forgotten that sleep existed. I somehow was able to replace sleep with food, at least for a while. And I talked to her. We could move her in a wheelchair. Months later, she could walk on crutches. She relearned all her cognitive capabilities from before, and then even some more.

Three years later, she had another episode, less severe. One young resident physician later became a student of mine, and he now applies my teachings as an additional tool to help his chronic pain patients.

Vanessa recovered. She speaks seven languages, holds three bachelor's degrees, and has two master's degrees in International Law. Physically, she has no residual damage. She is a happy, extraordinarily intelligent, exceedingly determined – I do not call it stubborn anymore – humanitarian woman.

Little did they know...

The scientific part of my brain needed to understand what had saved her. I still love science. Science and research are very important. But there is also a much stronger power, a power we cannot grasp yet. Even though we cannot fully understand and explain it, this power exists.

I studied like crazy. We had huge money troubles. No wonder with all the medical bills! I spent all money I could come up with and more than that on my studies. I needed to find out. I obsessively needed to figure it out. With hindsight, I learned it was hypnosis. I instinctively had worked with her higher mind! I took many certification classes with various teachers in numerous fields, intensified my background of alternative medicine including ancient healing modalities, and also became an OMNI Hypnosis Certification Instructor. OMNI Hypnosis is a specific hypnosis method established by Jerry Kein in Florida in 1979. The OMNI Hypnosis Training Center® International is now owned by Hansruedi Wipf, Switzerland, and is the very first hypnosis process worldwide that is ISO 9001 certified.

I made a very conscious, meaningful, and remarkable decision: I stopped limiting myself to the use of only my left brain, my analytical thinking part, and broadened my horizon by adding the use of my right brain, my emotional intuitive part. I left corporate to heal the world. Jerry Kein, one of my greatest teachers, encouraged me from day one on my new path to accept my purpose and to teach hypnosis. Jerry, I miss you. Jerry, I adore you.

So far, I have helped thousands of clients to create their small and giant miracles. I know, I know it, I *know* it's possible!

Allow me to lay out a road map for you, a path which may help you to navigate your challenging situation with certainty and in companionship. Let us align our compass and go step by step, steadily, unflinchingly, in the direction of your miracle.

You will see the importance of holding the reins of your life or taking them back. You, as a human being, are more than your body. Please consider your entire, complex entity. We will have a very close look to the magical power of your mind and how you can tap into your highest positive power. Chapter 3 will provide you with information about the concept of the four compartments of the "system man" and how to keep the entire system in balance or reestablish balance. The combination of those elements, applying the tools hand in hand and not isolated from each other, leads you closer and closer to your own miracle, to overcome your devastating diagnosis. It gives you the structure for your script of hope.

A brutally honest assessment of your situation is a prerequisite for a successful journey. That is what we will do in Chapter 4, and I will share with you a case study from my practice that gives proof for my statement, "Facts matter – Mind matters most." We need to know the facts first, before we can work on them, before we can change them. How to deal with change and get the best results through change will be discussed as well.

In the next chapter, you will experience how you can use your voice wisely. I will lead you through an exercise to restore or to practice speaking your truth. By the end of Chapter 5, you will understand why it is crucial to stand your ground, to speak your truth, and to be aware of your way of talking to yourself – all in high respect, politeness, and with certainty and love. We will also focus on hypnosis. I will explain how hypnosis works and what hypnosis can do for you. It is a natural state of the mind, and I invite you devotedly to discover that power portal for you and use it to your best possible benefit.

Stress and its symptoms, such as not enough sleep, are far-reaching topics which we will tackle in Chapter 6. I will give you exercises and explanations to help you to restore balance and develop a healthy sleep pattern again. When put into action, it will enable you to establish a modified relationship with stress and to create stress-levels for you which you can steer and handle.

Chapter 7 is going to be devoted to love and fear, their occurrence, their competition, and how you can combat the predominance of either fear or love. I will share with you exercises and models to make it easy to understand where imbalances come from and how you can reestablish a well-adjusted proportion of these complementary components.

The power of your mind, precisely guided by the right words, will lead you to great pain relief. You might find a deeper understanding of the purpose of pain and discover that pain actually is not only bad. It has a very important warning function. The conscious, purposeful use of the incredible capabilities of all levels of the mind will be an enormous help for you to manage that pain. I will show you methods to be the master of your brain. The vicious cycle of pain-feeds-suffering-feeds-pain needs to be broken, and you can do that. In Chapter 8, I will share with you how.

The next chapter provides you with the Golden Ticket, I will explain what I mean by that. We will have a heartfelt conversation. I really hope you will join me and share your thoughts about intuition, forgiveness, the struggles around forgiveness, and its incomparable healing power. We will exchange some thoughts about self-image and self-worth, and we will dare to embrace self-forgiveness, the high art of making peace.

Furthermore, we will examine the distinctions of information, knowledge, science and wisdom and how they build on and complement each other. Western Medicine and alternative treatments, energy healing techniques, and chemical substances all have their benefits. I am a passionate advocate for applying them all in a complementary, respectful way and recognizing their specific values. We need balance to be at peace. To create balance, we need an open mind. With an open mind, we have to face all aspects of the world and the individuum. We have to face both wolves. Allow me to introduce you to the two wolves in chapter 10.

In Chapter 11, we will accompany Stella on her preparation for her final act. She grants us unconcealed insights to her last journey and into her soul's travels. We will talk about sex. We will talk about the concept of lifetime contracts and graduation. And I will reveal why I am writing this book and open my innermost vulnerable core to you. Let us travel together with respect, compassion, and gentleness.

When the inevitable last journey has to be taken, when it is finally time to embark onto the next level, love is the most precious, most beautiful gift we all can offer. Chapter 12 is dedicated to advice and guidance for you, your loved ones, and anyone who might be involved in some way in this transition. I will share cases and experiences from my practice. I wholeheartedly wish that sharing those will soothe your fears, diminish your potential uncertainties, and give you guidance, strength, faith, and hope. Love is the most important thing in life, from the very beginning till the very end. It is all about love.

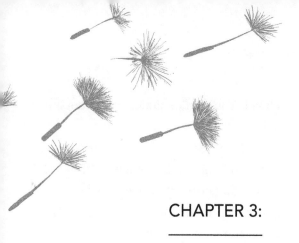

CHAPTER 3

Take the Driver's Seat

*"Life is like riding a bicycle. To keep your
balance, you must keep moving."*
– Albert Einstein

Take a deep breath. And another one, and maybe a third one. Keep breathing.

Now let's have a look what these shared stories have to do with *you*. You are possibly reading this book because you or someone you love is currently struggling with life, is confronted with a terminal diagnosis, or even has to face death very soon. Maybe you have to cope with a loss, and you strain yourself to fill the void.

It is a rough time, no doubt, no playing it down. But some tools, exercises, and strategies can help you in a big way to sustain those challenges a little more easily. We can do this hand in hand. You are not alone, even though it might feel very lonely.

I do see a human being as a complex structure consisting of four major compartments. To me, the "system man" is composed of body, mind, spirit, and soul. Every component has its own function. The soul is the home of our emotional learning and growing. It is the part of our being that creates and knows. Spirit communicates with us via our spiritual department. Spirit chooses and guides us. The mind accommodates our intellectual learning, thinking, and studying, and it develops patterns. And the body holds and shapes our physical being.

If all those segments are in balance, and when all divisions of the system communicate smoothly with each other, then we are healthy and feel fantastic. In the event of any disturbance in the communication between these elements or any imbalance within at least one part of the system, we need to get alarmed. How does this alarm system work? No matter where the imbalance occurs, the body is the part that gives the signals we can detect. The body speaks a language we can understand.

If you have a broken leg due to a physical injury, you would see a physician and get your leg fixed. If you have a small cut in your skin because you worked in the garden today, you would get a Band-Aid. When you have a headache, well, you can either ignore it or take a pill or listen to the underlying message. Sometimes the headache goes away. Sometimes it gets worse, and it is inevitable that your body tries to find a way to deliver an important message to you. Some messages require a signature upon delivery; some messages *need* to be received. The sooner we understand the hidden message, the better we can support our system to find balance. The very moment we understand the message, we understand the real cause of the issue. Then the body's job to tell us something is done, and the body is allowed to heal, to restore stability. The headache is substitutional for any other discomfort or sickness. Being in balance means to be sound. To restore balance is to enact the healing process. This can result in returning to health and purposeful living after a severe illness or in establishing peace for a fearless transition in love and pleasant anticipation to grow. Both are healing, both are a miracle.

In order to navigate this challenging time in the best way, we have to address several hazard zones (e.g. sleep, nutrition, emotional roller coasters, pain, and grief).

You need to be able to sleep despite stress and worries. It is crucial to recharge. The exercises I will teach you are highly efficient and easy to implement. With reliable methods to satisfactorily recharge your batteries, you can be more relaxed and use your energies wisely to master all troubles and hassles.

Nutrition and Exercise: Put the Plan into Action

Eating healthy and exercising are other cornerstones to restoring a balanced state. It is important to find out which foods are really good for you and which don't give you the best nourishment in your specific situation right now. It is imperative to draw up a fitness schedule tailor-made for you. Holding on to physical mobility according your condition very much supports your emotional resilience. But it is even more important to actually apply these grandiose food and workout plans to your daily routine as much as possible to obtain wellness.

Roller Coaster of Emotions: Take Back Control

What to do when the roller coaster of your irrepressible emotions starts again? It is absolutely okay to feel the total 360° circle of emotions colorfully, with all its highest highs and lowest lows. It is not okay to get stuck with your head in the sand. It is crucial to recognize your emotions, to address them, and to control them. Controlling your emotions does not equal suppressing them. To control the emotions means to be in control of your emotions, not the other way around. The moment when you gain back your control, when you are in charge, when you are the boss that is the moment when you open your gateway to healing. That is the moment when you live your life consciously and purposefully.

Pain Management: Manage That Pain

A basic prerequisite of living your life actively is being free of debilitating discomfort. Pain, physical or emotional, can drain your energy level dramatically. It has a huge effect on your mood, your appetite, and your enjoyment of life. To be able to participate in the delights of life, you need to manage the pain. An embedded, super effective, unfailing pain management system helps to afford a self-determined lifestyle. Pain management should not be limited to medical drugs. Chemicals are a good help and support, but we as living beings have an equally effective system available within us, within our mind. Our mind is the most powerful healer (or the opposite, a hefty destroyer) that I know. Pain is a symptom, a warning sign, a way for our body to communicate and hand us the information. We need to be able to feel pain in order to receive the message. What we do not need is to suffer in endless agony.

Truth Heals: Speak Your Truth

Most if not all of us long for a self-determined approach to life. It's our birthright to be the director of our own life. This, of course, has to be adjusted to our circumstances and our capabilities. For sure, this includes consideration and tactfulness for our families, caregivers, and all involved individuals. There is a huge difference between selfishness and self-worth. I do not advocate for any kind of selfish behavior, but I do encourage you to represent your sense of self-worth. To be able to point out what you really want, you need to know it first for yourself. Many of my clients are not aware of their deepest wishes. Many of my clients have never done this self-assessment before. It is a tremendous responsibility of yours to learn about your own desires. Only when you know what you really want, you can reveal your needs and wishes, and you can guide your assistants to provide you with the most supportive help possible, which in the end leads to fulfillment and contentment for all. It is your journey; it's about you. Tap into your inner mind. Don't be scared to figure things out about yourself. Truth heals. Find your truth, speak your truth, use the power of your mind, use your inner wisdom, and dissolve all fear.

Death Is Not the Ultimate End: Resolve Your Fear

Death, in our society, is often a very hushed-up matter. Death is treated as a taboo, yet we know it happens to all of us eventually. Death usually lives in very close relationship with fear and, as a result of that fear, also uncertainty. We do not know exactly, when death is going to visit or how it will knock. We very often feel unassertive in assisting someone in the process of dying and also, after the transition has happened, in encounters with the bereaved. It is extremely close to my heart to demystify death and dying. I grew up with the belief that death is the ultimate end that nobody makes it back from. That is why nobody could report about The End, the final act. It made sense to me and scared me, honestly. It made me freak out internally. The unknown was terrifying to me. I know that people make it back. There are living human beings who came back from heaven. Fear is a monster. Fear drags us down from flying high in understanding the Universe.

People who made it back usually don't talk about it because of fear – just like I didn't. I suspected that people would laugh at me, would reject me, or, even worse, would think I went crazy and would institutionalize me. With courage, I now tell you that I do not fear death anymore, not at all. After my NDEs (near death experiences) and multiple OBEs (out of body experiences), I feel no fear; I feel safe and awaited. I have, apart from some occasional attacks of homesickness, no yearning for the other side yet because I now know at least parts of my purpose and have accepted my mandate. My aim is to fulfill my assignment, to enjoy life gratefully, and later to soar fearlessly to the next level of growing. I wholeheartedly wish the same for you. Resolve all fear. Give yourself permission to freely embrace all challenges and joys in all stages of your journey called life. You deserve to feel safe because you are.

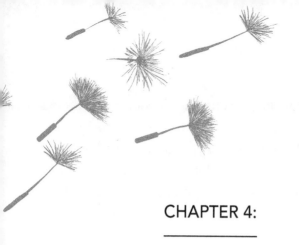

CHAPTER 4:

Facts Matter, Mind Matters Most

"It is such a mysterious place, the land of tears."
– Antoine de Saint-Exupéry

The more you know about your arcane wishes, the better you listen to your inner whisper, the more precise you can be with your utmost significant dreams and the more realistic it becomes to meet your goals. It is essential to establish a detailed roadmap to guide you out of the murky jungle of the tentacles of fear and despair up to the illuminating hills of assurance and security. I invite you to take stock now. Have a pure, unbiased, mercilessly honest look at your current situation. Face your deepest wishes and your boldest, king-sized dreams. The result of your analysis might be surprising to you. If you do this comprehensively and boundlessly while listening to your heart, you will find aspects of you and your circumstances which you haven't seen before. This will open a new perspective for you. By shifting the angle of your outlook, you will lead yourself to more self-determination and peace of mind.

*****

Assessment of Your Current Life-Situation

Area of Assessment	My Current Situation (you fill in)	Example Answers (based on Stella)
My diagnosis		Lung cancer, Stage 4
My treatments		Drs. A, B, C…; Hospitals X, Y, Z…; chemotherapy (x cycles, with y therapies), radiation; acupuncture, kinesiology; meditation, essential oils, crystals
Results of my treatment today		Decelerated growth of tumor; generation of metastasis; slightly enhanced condition and feeling

Second opinions		Dr. D, Dr. E; naturopath, holistic treatment center
Alternative treatment options (not used yet)		Hypnosis, energy healing, Shamanic healing methods, Angelic healing modalities
My support system in place		Partner, child/children, extended family, friends, neighbors, social network, colleagues, nursing service
My additional support options		Cleaning service; meals on wheels, grocery shopping online; driving service; homework help for kids; hairdresser home service
My biggest struggles		Fear, fear of pain; sleep; asking for help, receiving help; how to control my innermost feelings; how to transition

My deepest, heartfelt wishes		One year to live in good quality; romantic intimate time with my husband; time and courage to talk with my children about my passing; fearless, self-determined transition; being loved until my earthly end; being able to show my love as long as I live; to actively steer my final act
My options to find help to create my own, unique miracle		Husband, children; coach; hypnosis

*****

Congratulations! After taking the time and guts to fill out your assessment, please honor yourself and your courage and allow yourself to feel proud. This is a remarkably difficult task that you just tackled. Do not underestimate the importance of that step on your pathway to inner peace. Your statements are the partitura for your *concerto grosso*. Your orchestra consists of varicolored instruments. You have many different option, various methods and treatment modalities at hand. You belong on the conductor's rostrum. You beat time. You conduct.

Accept your position in your life. It is the driver's seat! Never ever think you dream too big – never, never, never.

Big dreams are the stuff miracles are made of. Never underestimate the power of your mind.

Modern Science Teamed Up with Complimentary Medicine

Modern science seems to agree that every single illness has at least one share of emotional impact. Over time, emotional perceptions can lead to physical symptoms. If your body has created physical symptoms to raise your awareness for a specific problem, the most successful way to solve this issue is to treat you as a whole entity. It is not sufficient to just treat the symptoms. We need to find the cause of your issue and solve that problem at the root. The holistic approach, the overall cooperation of diverse experts, very often results in the best possible outcome. Trust the knowledge of the experts. Seek the help of multiple domains and weave your dazzling web of miracles.

Through my practice, I've learned that people receive outstanding treatment for their physical body. I give high credit to science and medicine. But that is not enough from my point of view. The mind, soul, and spiritual level are also components of a human being and deserve to be considered as well. We create what we think. What we can imagine becomes our reality. When you know how to guide your mind, when you consistently and precisely instruct your mind to do what you really want, then you are the architect of your miracle. Let me share with you an incredible example of the immeasurable, fascinating power of the mind.

The Mind Overwrites the Body

My client Marc sought out my services because of *Kinderwunsch* (desire to have children). He is happily married, and he and his wife had tried everything. They have been together for more than ten years, and after five years of verifying whether they would love to spend the rest of their lives as a married couple, they exchanged vows, rings, and kisses. From then on, she could not suppress her *Kinderwunsch* any longer. Marc was pretty relaxed during the first months of trying to make a baby. Sure, he wanted to manifest his love for his beautiful wife with a baby, too. However, in the beginning of their journey to become parents, his desire was not as burning as hers. After some unsuccessful months he became nervous and it started to scratch his ego. Following a time of real concerns about their fertility and dramatically increasing emotional pain for his wife, Marc realized how much he wished to have a baby with his amazing wife. Marc wanted to make his wife happy, and he intended to be a loving, caring dad. After two years of constant swinging between hope and disappointment, they agreed to consult a specialist. The urologist found lowered levels of testosterone and prescribed external testosterone to kick-start his manhood. His wife's results proved all to be in optimum range. Higher hopes were followed by deeper falls month after month. This became their routine. Due to his low sperm quality, they were transferred to the *Kinderwunsch* clinic with the best reputation. According to her menstrual cycle, they started to prepare for insemination. The date was set, and with excitement and euphoria, they were waiting for that day. He gave his sperm sample, and later that same day, she would conceive. That was the plan. Instead of having the procedure done, she was informed that there was nothing they could work with. Nothing! Shock! In their desperation, he gave another sample, but the time of hope was short. The shattering result was confirmed. Nothing. Zero. Null. Tears, silence, and self-pity followed by anger occupied the couple's days. They could not avoid feeling the pain of grief.

Phases of Grief: Change Management

According to findings of Dr. Elisabeth Kübler-Ross, grief consists of five phases. These are: denial, anger, bargaining, depression, and acceptance. Although I absolutely agree to those phases, I mostly experience that, with my clients, the order is different. After the shock of the news, almost all of them go into denial. For the majority of my clients, the next phase is bargaining. This one is followed by anger. The phase of depression, the phase of deep, deep sadness migrates into acceptance and allows them to rebuild a sense of peace and an outlook on life including making plans for the future. The stages do not always show up isolated. They can overlap and be interwoven. It is essential to progress through *all* of them. Any hold-ups hinder healing and peace. This way, emotional wounds tend to build less scar tissue. The same phases can be observed in any change management process.

Strategies of Change Management

Marc's wife was tired, exhausted from seeing her fundamental dream partially dying each month. She tried to fill the void with sweet comfort. Sugar was the only thing she could think of to hush the screaming emptiness. Because her self-worth was almost dissolved, she didn't really care about her increasing weight and her decreasing constitution. She went to work, teaching school kids with unbowed enthusiasm. This was her coping mechanism. She put all her love towards other people's children. She suffered silently.

Marc chose a different strategy. His motivation was his wife. He was committed to keeping his promise; he wanted to make her happy. Marc changed his diet. Both had gained a lot of weight during these years of emotional roller coaster. Now he wanted to restore his original fitness. He implemented a workout routine again and stopped drinking alcohol completely. Although they had consulted another world-renowned fertility center and although his results had been negligibly better, they had to hear the knockdown summary: "You will never become biological parents naturally."

Working with a Coach and Hypnotist

Marc was ready to move heaven and earth. In his mind's eye, he could see them having children. He had dropped many pounds, was eating healthy food, exercised regularly, had a good sleep routine and was successful at his executive job. Regardless of the challenges which the last five years of regular monthly frustration had provided, regardless of the bruises and scratches their marriage had been hurt with, the couple was able to maintain a firm, trusting relationship. Marc had retrieved some self-esteem and was ready to trust the power of his mind. The Universe had managed to pave the way for him. Less than thirty minutes prior to Marc's call for an appointment, a client had to reschedule, and I could offer him the opening. His co-workers at a famous Swiss bank stepped into the breach and enabled Marc to take advantage of the offer.

On May 5th, we had our first session. His wife had given up hope; she did not want to restart the hurtful cycle.

We conducted an intense session, started the engines. After explaining what hypnosis is, how it works, and what hypnosis can do for him, I guided Marc into this natural state of mind. I helped him to regress back to the initial event that caused his issue. Marc drifted back in the submerged memories of his childhood. At the early age of four, his subconscious mind took one sentence said to him too literally and challenged his manhood. We easily could correct this misunderstanding. We released this false imprint and replaced it by a new, desired one.

Marc was given a bunch of homework, easy yet powerful exercises for his mind, to solidify the newly made imprint. With the intent to lift the heaviness of the term "homework" - work is often associated with feelings of strain and dissatisfaction - I rather prefer to call it home-fun because working with your mind can be really fun and very fulfilling. We also established a plan for his follow-up tests of his sperm-quality and for our next meeting. Human male sperms need sixty-four days to complete maturity. Therefore, we rearranged his schedule for check-ups on his sperm-numbers from every four weeks to 128 days plus. I wanted him to have enough time to have at least two full cycles for his sperms to develop. His results in September were promising but still not sky-high, yet much higher than sea-level. We continued with our program, and Marc's commitment was even more stimulated by the pleasing results. Another minimum of 128 days would give him plenty of time to apply his new tools and build towards their dream. A third session was dedicated to his wife, and we worked vicariously on her, as a matter of course with her permission which we received prior to our work.

According to his schedule, I expected his new results in December. Marc did not call in December; I was not concerned about it. I assigned it to the holidays.

The work we do, the work with the mind, is very personal, and I consider it a work based on trust. If you do not trust your hypnotist, do not work with this particular hypnotist. If you do not trust your therapist, stop working with your therapist. In my opinion, the same holds true for medical professionals of any field. It definitely goes in both directions.

In January of the following year, he called as promised. To my surprise, he had not showed up for his next test, so there was no data for me and my analytical mind. Instead, he disclosed his wife's pregnancy. Oh, what compelling news for my emotional brain and my compassionate heart! What a joy! What a miracle! They had to overcome five years of lost hope, suffering, treatments, spending tremendous amounts of money, and shedding oceans of tears. After only another eight months and three sessions on working with the super powerful mind, they were expecting. No doubts – it is his baby. Their pregnancy was overall a smooth one and abundantly filled with pleasant anticipation and happiness and love. Nine months later in September, she gave birth naturally to their healthy, long desired baby. The lesson learned for Marc and his family: Never lose your belief! Always have faith! You will be rewarded in the end. Marc and his wife now have their divine reward, their precious baby boy. They created their miracle.

The beginning of life and the end of it are very close to each other. Both are transitions to the next level of being, which include a lot of learning. The unknown is what scares us. The case of Marc, his wife, and their son is a case of tremendous pain, deep grief, and indescribable thankfulness. It gives proof of the undreamed-of power of the mind. The mind is capable of solving physical limitations beyond our wildest grasp. Working with the mind makes miracles become reality, no matter whether it is about entering life or leaving this lifetime. The mind, when guided precisely and trusted with its power, gives us peace and fulfillment. We only need to trust. I think this is one of the biggest tasks in life. It starts with trusting ourselves, trusting the power of our own mind.

CHAPTER 5:

Truth Heals

"Unthinking respect for authority is the greatest enemy of truth."
– Albert Einstein

Jacob called with a very weary voice. He hesitantly asked for an appointment. Jacob was not sure if anything in the world could help him scramble out of this desperate situation nor if it would make any sense to keep trying. He was even more in doubt as I told him, "Yes, that is possible for sure, but you are the only one who can get you out of there. I definitely can help you, but I cannot do it for you. I will accompany you. I will guide you. I will cheer you up. I will have your back, and I will celebrate with you. Are you willing to do your part? I am entirely committed to contributing my piece." Maybe because of my assurance, he signed up to work with me.

Jacob, in his late 50's, hiding behind a well-tended beard, impassively answered my questions during the intake. He was married and has one grown-up daughter. He suffered an early loss of an adult brother. Jacob was self-employed, wrongfully accused of having caused an accident. He had no chance to prove his innocence. The involvement in the resulting deposition was the straw that broke the camel's back. He was ineffably overwhelmed by life. Bookkeeping. Property maintenance. Sleep deprivation. Overweight. All he saw were obligations. Jacob thought he was a disappointment to all his loved ones. He felt like he was a burden. He did not want to be a burden, and he did not want to carry his burden any longer.

We were taking inventory. We gently pulled the veil aside to give him a glimpse of his dusty dreams. They had not been nurtured and polished for a long time, but they were still there. I could draw his interest, and he tentatively engaged.

As I had explained to Stella and Marc and all my clients, I illustrated to Jacob how the mind works, which I adapted from Jerry F. Kein's Mind Model. I wanted to show him how he could tap into the various levels of his miraculous mind and awaken his dreams to life. His lethargy transmuted into fidgeting. Jacob had a hard time controlling his frame of mind. Upon his approval, I decided to give him a little calming exercise based on an idea of Dr. Arthur Winkler.

It is good practice that I really like. Please join Jacob and me and participate.

Advice

My valued reader, I suggest that you do not close your eyes right now. Please give your mind permission to be carried away into a wonderful state of relaxation whilst you are reading these soothing words. Maybe you choose to ask someone to read it to you. Alternatively, you can read it out loud and record it so that you can listen to the words over and over again with your eyes closed. Or allow me to present you with the calming effect of water when you decide to work with me.

Exercise: Water

*****

Please sit comfortably and take a deep breath. Hold it for a moment and with your exhale, relax your body and your mind. Focus on your breathing and continue breathing gently. When you are ready, no later than with your third exhale, close your eyes. Concentrate on your eyelids and relax your eyelids as much as you can. Relax them completely. Now you can expand this quality of relaxation over your whole body.

Now we are going to give your subconscious mind a signal. This signal will cause you to become calm and relaxed on your wish. The unconscious levels of your mind will cause the signal to work.

From now on for the rest of your life, whenever you wish, every time you look at water, the unconscious levels of your mind and all levels of your inner mind will cooperate and cause you to become relaxed, calm, and peaceful. Every time you look at water, your nerves become more relaxed and steadier, and you continue becoming calmer emotionally. Any water you look at is an automatic signal, including rain, puddles of water, water coming out of a faucet, water in a shower or bathtub, water in a swimming pool, a pond, a creek, a river, a lake, in the ocean, or in a bottle or glass.

Being calmer and more relaxed enables you to think more clearly. It enables you to focus your attention more readily. You will be able to better concentrate. That causes your memory to keep improving. You will also find that being more calm and relaxed causes all of your body processes and activities to continue functioning more perfectly, and that causes your health and mood to keep improving each day. You will be pleased to find yourself experiencing many other really wonderful benefits.

From now on for the rest of your life, when you wish to, every time you look at water, your mind will cause you to become relaxed, calm, and feel very peaceful, and you will remain that way as you go about your daily activities. You will have more energy, more strength and vitality, and you will continue becoming more efficient in your work and other activities from being more relaxed and more at ease.

I will be counting from one to three, and by the number of three, not before, you will be back in the here and now, back in the present moment, opening your eyes and feeling calm, relaxed, and at peace.

1. Take a deep breath and let a wave of joy ripple through your body.

2. Take another deep breath, move your fingers and your toes, stretch.

3. Open your eyes, feeling great, much better than before.

How do you feel? Do you notice how calm you are? That is great, isn't it?

*****

For Jacob, he is now beautifully relaxed and focused. Now he is ready to absorb my explanation of hypnosis. It is a very simplified, abstract illustration. I am convinced when you understand how hypnosis works, then you will know that it is an absolutely natural state of the mind. We experience hypnosis at least twice a day. Just before we become fully awake – fully aware of the day – and before we fall asleep. These passages, this trance-like state, is hypnosis. Deliberately entering this relaxed yet highly focused state is hypnosis.

Meditation - Prayer - Hypnosis

With the intent to shake off the misconceptions and dissolve all the baseless fears about hypnosis, I came up with a concrete, easy-to-grasp characterization:

To me, we immerse into the similar state of mind when we say prayers, meditate, or become hypnotized. The differences I see are in the purpose of the activities:

Through prayers, we ask for something (help, guidance, protection, peace, health, for us and for others); we surrender.

With meditation, we slow down the traffic of our own thoughts to the point that the noisy chit-chat becomes quiet enough that we can hear (ideas, notions, perspectives, epiphanies). When we meditate, we listen.

In hypnosis, we work on something. We systematically use this highly concentrated state of mind to achieve something, to change something (habits, perspectives, bodily issues, emotional problems). We are an active transformer.

Hypnosis: How Does It Work?

The Conscious Mind

As hypnotists, we imagine our brain symbolically consisting of three layers. The outside layer represents the conscious mind. In the conscious mind, all analytical thinking takes place, all the logic, all judgement. Our short-term memory is also located in this level of the mind. All the information we access frequently, e.g. how to brush your teeth, how to use the light-switch, your route to work are stored in the short-term memory. The conscious mind also accommodates our will power when you make a decision, such as "I stop worrying constantly." This is a decision you make with your conscious mind, in the outside layer of the brain and only there.

The Subconscious Mind

One layer deeper in the brain, our subconscious mind resides. The subconscious mind is the home of all our emotions, our feelings, the home of our habits and patterns, as well as our long-term memory and processes for self-preservation. Self-protection makes sure that you are always safe. You are always in control. I like to imagine the long-term memory as a huge library which stores everything what we have experienced with all our five senses – sight, hearing, touch, taste, smell. Whenever we need specific information, for instance when we want to find the cause of a problem, we can enter our permanent memory in the subconscious mind and find out about everything we need to know at this specific time, for this specific topic, for this specific issue. In the hypnotic state, we can discern the cause of a problem, can release it, and restore balance. The solution is within you. The solution is in your inner mind, and you can operate your mind wisely to regain control of your life, tapping into your own infinite wisdom will facilitate your healing, your finding balance and peace.

The Unconscious Mind

On the inside of the layer system of the brain is our unconscious mind. The unconscious mind is responsible for all automatic bodily functions, like cell division, immune system operations, blood pressure, breath rate, heart rate, and blood sugar regulation – all the things that are happening whether we think about them or not. While we are asleep, we breathe; our heart beats. It doesn't matter whether we consciously take care of it. It just happens.

The Protective System

To prevent that every information can assimilate into the subconscious mind unhindered, uncontrolled, we develop a guard, the critical factor. In our early childhood years, this protective system is not established yet, and all data are embedded in the subconscious mind. Our guard restrictively allows only certain information to pass the gate, only the "truth" goes through. The truth is what is programmed within the subconscious mind. In case you want to change your programming, you need to bypass that critical guard to configure your new truth. That is exactly what we can achieve with hypnosis. Hypnosis is the bypassing of the critical factor and the establishment of acceptable, selective thinking. Hypnosis is a trance-like state, in which you have heightened focus and concentration.

You are Always in Control

Every single hypnosis is self-hypnosis. Nobody can force you into hypnosis. The hypnotist is just your manual. Please always remember: Every single hypnosis is self-hypnosis. I am your tour guide. I like to compare a hypnosis session with a walk to the top of a mountain. We climb jointly. We are a team.

Another image to understand hypnosis is to picture the mind as a gearbox. The different levels of the mind are represented by separate gears. When we imagine the conscious mind as one cogwheel and the subconscious mind as a second one, then it is crucial to have both parts taken care off, to have both gear-wheels in very good and clean shape and engage them, bring them together. That way, the car can run smoothly.

Jacob was very familiar with trucks and mechanics and gears. It clicked, and his concerns were dissolved.

I am certain that our brain is a huge gift for us and that we use just a tiny amount of the capacity our brain has to offer.

Let us use as much of our brain as possible. Let us engage analysis and emotions; let us take care of the balance in life.

Stand Your Ground and Use Your Voice

Besides taking inventory (see Chapter 4: Assessment of Your Current Life Situation) it is very important to speak up for yourself, for your innermost wishes, and for the things which are not good for you.

Jacob had a very hard time connecting with his emotions. He had built a wall around his heart. Feeling his emotions was too painful for him. Unconsciously, he had created a protective shield around his heart. This wall prevented him from being hurt; it numbed the pain. At the same time, it also numbed every other, every positive feeling. For a very long time, he was able to cope with life that way. He had cut off his feelings like an unwanted limb. Now it was time for him to become whole again. Jacob's dream was to find joy in life again. Otherwise…

To live his dream, he needed to be able to stand up for himself against this unfair accusation that had led to the deposition on the horizon. Who knew what else might follow in this process? His worries were gigantic and omnipresent. To be able to speak your truth, you first need to become aware of your deepest inner truth, your deepest feelings, biggest concerns, and boldest wishes and dreams. Jacob knew deep inside he wanted to live. He wanted to be happy and free from dark moods. It was really tough for him to say it out loud: "I can do this."

I shared with Jacob – and I invite you to participate with him – the following exercise:

Exercise: Throat

*****

Stand with your legs shoulder-width apart. (If this is not possible for you, any other position is okay as well. It is just more profound to feel the difference when you can stand.) Gently put your open hand on your throat and cover your neck. Say out loud something you know for sure is your truth. For instance, say your name and feel the vibration. "My name is Jacob." Now slowly, in small steps, let your hand slide down with your palm pressed on the front of your body. Continuously repeat your sentence out loud, and notice your vibration. How far down can you feel it vibrating? Can you feel it in your hand at the whole chest area? Ideally you can feel it down to the breastbone.

Now choose a sentence, which is not your truth. I asked Jacob to say, "My name is Petra." Repeat the sequence. How far down are you able to detect a vibration now? Do you recognize that the vibration stops very far up, close to the throat?

Now say something you are not sure about whether you can do it. When you know this is your truth, practice saying it. Use your hand and repeat your truth-statement until you can feel the vibration down to your breastbone.

Notice how good it feels to be in sync with yourself. Commemorate how wonderful it feels to be in harmony.

*****

This exercise is incredibly helpful to tune in to your inner power. It will enable you to communicate your inner wishes with grace and confidence. It's very important to communicate clearly with everyone including for instance your loved ones, your medical professionals, your co-workers, your friends, and most importantly yourself. When you admit what you really want and what you don't want, it is much easier to find the right words and a polite tone to transmit your message and build on your dream. It makes it easier for the people who care for you to fulfill your wishes and needs because they know what you really want when you tell them. They do not have to guess. You help to make it clear and easy for all parties involved when you speak up for yourself. This is most efficient when you communicate honestly, precisely and respectfully. No matter in which phase of your life you are, clear, honest, respectful communication is key. It starts within.

Admit if something is not good for you. I am not talking about nagging, I am referring to something that is important to you, something that compels you to dwell on it. Do not diminish it by simply saying "It's okay" when it is not okay. You need to acknowledge it to be able to change it. Before you can restore balance, you need to be aware that something went off-kilter. There might be no chance to change the circumstances, but you always have the chance to change how you navigate it. You can always change your perspective and your attitude.

How Do You Talk to Yourself?

How is your internal communication? How do you start your day? What is the first thing you say to yourself? What are the last words at the end of each day you say to yourself? How many times a day do you talk yourself down? How do you talk to the wonderful person you are? Can you see the beauty in you? Can you see yourself as the whole entity? Can you see your beautiful soul? Better be nice to yourself. Stop negative self-talk. Immediately. I suggest starting your day with a kind, loving greeting. "Good morning, gorgeous" or "Good morning, handsome" are sincere words to start the day with. Please test it. Accept the challenge and greet yourself every single morning for at least thirty consecutive days with those loving words. I promise, you will feel the difference. I am your guinea pig. Many years ago, I was in my early twenties, a very well-meaning lady requested me to do this. Hesitantly, I obeyed her advice. It worked and still does; it became part of my morning ritual. This is how you set yourself up for the day. This sets the energy for how you will communicate with others. By the end of each day, say something for which you are grateful the day has given to you and caringly, tenderly, lovingly wish yourself a restful "Good night, beautiful soul."

Stella was very nice in talking about her family. Loving words in gentle tone left her mouth when she was narrating about her loved ones. For herself, she had a deprecative hand movement, escorted by harsh words of discontentment. We changed how she talked to and about herself, and almost instantly, her tension eased, and she could bashfully start to receive compliments and affection from others.

For Jacob, it was essential to confess that this accusation scared him half to death, that it was tremendously unfair and really nasty. The perceived injustice of the situation revived him and his plea for his values.

In the moment, Marc could not pretend any longer that it was okay; he became brutally honest with himself and admitted the truth. He took charge of his/their life, reconnected with the power of his mind, and healed. Truth heals.

What is your inner truth? When you analyze your situation and compare it with your inner wishes, how much are they in sync? Do you sometimes silence yourself? Is it your desire to please others? Is it your feeling of not being worthy to consider some changes? Or is it your fear that you might not find the right tone and might hurt the people who care about you? Think twice, please. Wouldn't you be happy if others were honest and open with you? Wouldn't it be easier to fulfill other's expectations if you just knew about them? How rewarding is it for you to make your loved ones happy? Right, that is fulfilling and gives you joy as well. The same is true for the people who love you, the people who care for you. Make it as easy as you can for both sides. The situation is hard enough. Speak your truth. Use your voice, and if necessary, stand your ground. This is a major part of being in balance. Balance is the desired state of being. Balance is healing.

CHAPTER 6

Hush, Hush Beautiful Soul

"If you love a flower that lives on a star, it is sweet to look at the sky at night.
All the stars are a-bloom with flowers."

– Antoine de Saint-Exupéry

Balancing Your Energy-Level

By dissolving the inner attrition, you minimize friction. Incongruency between your inner and outer world created by not clearly announcing what you know and feel inside consumes a lot of energy. That is energy you really need and could make good use of. You patched a lingering leakage of valuable energy. You will recognize this in your energy levels, the shorter time you need to recharge, and the better quality of your recharge.

Stress and Its Symptoms

Stress is a commonly used term. A very high percentage of people feel stressed. Various studies in America, such as those done by the American Psychology Association and all over the world, show that people feel stressed about any kind of topic and the younger generations seem to have lower resistance to stress. This is for sure due to many different reasons. One factor might be that their parents feel more stressed already compared to their grandparents. If the youngsters cannot learn how to cope with stress, it is even harder for them. Stress became a very common state of being. To feel stressed is the new normal, and it is unquestionably accepted in our society.

Long-lasting stress can lead to physical, emotional, or cognitive symptoms. Symptoms such as low energy, higher heartbeat, high blood pressure, headaches, upset stomach, nausea, frequent colds, clenched jaw and grinding teeth, ringing in the ear, loss of sexual desire, loneliness, worthlessness, overwhelm, depression, being withdrawn, low self-esteem, frustration, agitation, mood swing, losing control, constant worrying, racing thoughts, forgetfulness, disorganization, lack of focus, pessimism, and poor judgement.

In a challenging life-situation, we get another thing on top of our already fully-loaded life. Have you or a loved one struggled with a terminal diagnosis? If yes, you most likely felt very stressed. That is normal. That is okay for a moment, your moment. Take the time you need to recognize it, accept it. Then take a deep breath and start your process of climbing out of this unserviceable state. It will be much easier when you see stress more as a state of mind than as an unscalable mountain in front of you.

In a medical or biological context, stress is a physical, mental, or emotional factor that causes bodily or mental tension (MedizinNet). Hans Seyle defined it in 1936 as "the non-specific response of the body to any demand for change." Originally, this term came up in Hooke's Law of 1658, the magnitude of an external force, or stress, produces a proportional amount of deformation, or strain, in a malleable metal." Hooke discovered the law of elasticity. The term stress was a physical one and became applied more and more over time on physiological similar responses. Stress is a more or less elastic response to pressure.

Disarm Stress

For me, stress in the context of life's challenges is a discrepancy between the task and the aptitude. I see stress as a gap, no more and no less.

When you have a task to fulfill and you know for sure you can do this easily, when you sense no gap between the job and your skills, you do not feel any kind of stress. You can just start to perform the duty. Let's say you are asked to write down your name, address, and phone number on a sheet of paper handed to you together with a pen, you probably can do this with ease and don't feel any stress.

If you are asked, as an example, to write down a very complicated quantum physics calculation, chances are much higher that you think you might not be able to solve this problem and feel stressed. (Of course, this is not the case for you if you are a quantum physicist).

We are constantly comparing what is asked of us and what we think we are capable of. If this is a match, fine. No stress. If there is a mismatch, if there is a gap, we feel stressed. Stress is a result of how we estimate our own capabilities in relation to the demands. If requirement and supply are equal, we are at ease; we are in balance. If the needs do not match the offers, if there is a gap, we are out of balance and feel stressed. Based on the need to feel balanced, we can create a state of being at ease. We also understand that for any chance of development, for any chance of improvement, we need that gap. Because we aspire to close the gap, we stretch ourselves and strive for more. For our brain, it is no difference which one, the task or our ability, is bigger or smaller; it is just the disproportion which creates the negative emotion. If we are permanently unchallenged, we feel bored, and over time we will experience similar symptoms as if we were constantly overwhelmed.

Decrease Your Stress: Close the Gap

Based on the imagery of stress being a gap, you can work on closing it.

You most likely cannot change a diagnosis, but maybe you can change how you feel about it. If you follow Mr. Seyle in thinking of stress as the response to the demand of change, you can steer your sentience. You can decrease the level of stress significantly when you increase the elasticity of your response and combine it with the process of change management.

What is your expectation for yourself? How high do you set the bar to be satisfied with your yield? Do you ever allow yourself to perform less than perfect? What is perfect for you?

With Stella, we investigate what her value system considers a necessity. She finds out that the only truly important thing for her is loving her family. This is – and she is absolutely sure – the one thing she is perfect at. Yes, she loves her family perfectly, no restraints. Wow! What a relief. There is no gap between her expectation and her reality. She feels the burden lifted. The most important thing in life is love. She is capable to fully love. The stress is getting smaller. We work our way through hundreds of less significant elements like cooking, cleaning, her doctor's appointments, decorating the house according to the seasons and so on. Together we develop a plan for Stella to find alternative ways to match expectation and objectivity. Stella readjusts her value system; she resets her priorities, and she opens up to asking for and accepting help.

Get help for things somebody else can do for you. Do not cut down on the thing only you can give. Love generously! There are many ways to show your love. Maybe you need to change the manner of showing your love due to your changed health condition and physical strength, but do not change or even stop to express your love.

Stella and I broke the big hazard called stress down into bite-size pieces and designed a tailormade system specifically adapted to her circumstances, which she can easily apply to her life. Gently but steadily, we closed the gap. Now Stella knows that she can handle any situation, any challenge with *grandeur*. The plan is great, and Stella can smile brightly and genuinely for a moment. But her eyes sadden, and she shares that the only issue was that she had real difficulties accepting help. Does this sound familiar to you?

Enable the Giver to Give by Receiving

This is very common. Many, if not most of us, think we are not worthy of receiving. Please step in the position of the other person, the one who wants to serve you. Just walk in the shoes of the giver for a moment. As the caregiver, you need someone to gift with your efforts. Nothing makes the servant's heart happier or more fulfilled than a serendipitous recipient feeling calm and comforted. Again, we need balance. For the giver to be able to give, they need a taker who is able to take. Only if both are willing to accept their position, the proverbial give and take is possible. The willing recipient is needed just as much as the donor.

Celebrate the Tiny Successes

Stella swallows dryly. She had never seen it from this perspective. Nobody likes to be rejected, not even the caregiver. Stella's mindset shifts, and she understands now that she is able to learn receiving for the giver's sake. As a second step, she commits to learning to receive because of herself. Yessss! This is huge! I am super excited and very proud of her. We celebrate Stella's revelation with a little silly dance. She is happy, smiling, radiant, calm, at peace. I think it is vital to celebrate, to feel, and express excitement in every single phase of our lives. No matter how tough the overall situation might be, every single tiny moment you feel joy is worth being savored.

Balancing Your Chakras

In order to make the important lesson of receiving easier to learn for her, I conduct a chakra-clearing. Chakras are energy centers inside and outside of our body. The word chakra is Sanskrit and means wheel. The chakras are supposed to spin smoothly and communicate clearly with each other. To allow your life force energy to flow freely and unhindered, there must not be any blocks of the chakras. With Stella, we focus on the seven chakras within her body. Chakras can sometimes become blocked through an emotional shock such as a devastating diagnosis. Therefore, I check Stella's chakras, cleanse them energetically, and bring them back to their natural swirl and reconnect them with each other. I use shamanic techniques of energy healing. Stella receives the energy with closed eyes and describes where in her body she feels the vortexes. It is amazing how intensely she feels the release of the blockages and the change in her energy system. Stella is beautifully relaxed, and her mind is working enormously without any effort. She is curious and asked tons of questions. My heart sings, and with pure joy, I share the ancient wisdom with her.

The Seven Chakras of the Physical Body

We start at the root chakra. It is located at the base of your spine. The root chakra's purpose is to connect you with Mother Earth, to make sure that you are grounded and to support and secure your survival here on earth. The corresponding color is red.

Next to the base chakra upwards comes the sacral chakra with the color orange, and it is located in your pelvic area. It is the center of pleasures, sexuality, and creativity.

Further up we find the solar plexus, the power center, the center of your self-esteem and your identity. Its matching color is yellow and it is located right above the belly button.

The heart chakra follows with the color green, and it is the home of your love, including self-love, and compassion. It is located in the breastbone area and is associated with health and healing.

The throat chakra is the fifth chakra and allows you to speak your truth with kindness. It resides between the collarbones and has a special connection to the color blue.

The sixth chakra is called the third eye. It is located between your eyebrows, exactly where the pineal gland resides in the middle of the brain. The little pineal gland is responsible for your day and night rhythm. It helps you to be awake during the day and sleep safe and sound at night. The third eye is able to receive information beyond the five senses. The third eye's correlating color is indigo.

The colors violet and white are linked to the seventh chakra, the crown chakra. It is located at the top of your head and builds the energetic bridge with the Universe. It is consciousness energy of individuality and universality. The crown chakra connects us with Father Sky like the root chakra connects us with Mother Earth.

Whilst we are talking and as I perform my energy clearing and balancing techniques, I give Stella suggestions for the colors to work with in the future to nurture her chakras.

Exercise: Rainbow

*****

Imagine the colors of the rainbow. With every breath you take, you can inhale all the colors of the rainbow. Your supply of all the colors is infinite. With every inhale, you send the exact amount of the exact matching color to your corresponding chakra, which receives the color gratefully, and you keep your chakras spinning and communicating perfectly fine with each other. The colors help you sustain beautiful balance and continuous healing.

*****

How to Improve Your Sleep

Stella feels very well-centered, steady, and completely in control now. She is ready to reestablish a high-quality sleep regime. She has not been able to get good quality sleep for sufficient hours or at the times she wants to fall asleep. Usually she sleeps for an hour or ninety minutes before worries, fear, anger, and pain wake her up again. Stella tries to get back to sleep, to be quiet in order to not wake up her family, and to not cry because she feels so lonely. She puts a lot of effort into her attempt but has not succeeded. She is chronically sleep deprived. Her tolerance is diminished, and she always feels guilty when she caught up on some sleep during the day. She thinks everyone else sustains a day without a nap. She, as the mother and the role model, is obligated to be hard working all day long. The magnitude of her frustration is constantly increasing, leading to more friction and arguments at home. It is time for a change!

You Deserve to Rest and Recharge

Many of us are raised with platitudes like "from nothing comes nothing," "whoever rests rusts," or "no pain, no gain". I agree to a certain extent. Hope and focused work are needed to be successful in any area of life. Only with good self-care and properly charged energy levels are we able to accomplish big and small things. To implement that, you might have to change your perspective. You might need to change some beliefs. The exercise I will share with you in a moment will help you calm down your spinning thoughts and guide yourself into a comfortable state of relaxation and a good sleep afterwards.

Please keep in mind, in case you are a parent, you are a role model. Yes, you teach your children your paradigm. Being active is one side of the coin. The other side is as important as being active. It is self-care. How you take care of yourself is what you pass on to your children. How do you want your children to care for themselves? Do you want them to eat unhealthy food on the fly? Do you want them to not rest? Do you want them to only work and not take the time to enjoy their accomplishments? No. Surely, not. Do you want them to feel guilty for recharging and gathering their vigor? Of course not. Please cut off all ties between guilt and recovery for good. You owe it to your loved ones and yourself to take good care of yourself. "There is no better medicine than sleep," my Mom used to say during my childhood years. It still sticks with me. Especially in a time of sickness, we need to provide our body, mind, and soul the time to recuperate, which is most effective during sleep. All other bodily functions are slowed down so that the body can invest as much energy as possible into restoring balance, into healing.

How to Hush Your Beautiful Soul

Now, how do you fall asleep on demand when your head is spinning around fear and worries? Hush your thoughts. Gently guide your head to rest so that your body can follow. Your thoughts are all over the place until you take the lead, until you climb into the driver's seat.

Dolphins sleep with just one half of their brain at a time. This enables them to continue breathing and not drown. They allow one side of the brain to sleep and keep the other half of their brain alert. They rest next to another dolphin; they rest in pairs. The second one puts his opposite side of the brain asleep. That works for them to observe their environment, to be able to detect any danger, and to get the adequate amount of sleep they need. Since it is not possible for us as human beings to share the task of sleeping between individuals or our brain partitions, we need to have our whole brain resting. It is important to become a master in calming your mind.

Focus on Your Breathing

For us, it is not possible to operate our brain hemispheres separately for sleep. We are lucky if we can control the speed of our stream of thoughts on demand. A powerful way to pilot your brain to calm down is to focus on breathing. You kindly but strictly focus all your thoughts on your breathing.

Exercise: Breathing

*****

To make this really easy, I suggest you create a mantra. This could be something like, "I am enough." Inhale and say out loud or silently, "I am," pause for a short moment, then exhale and say, "enough." Pause for a moment, repeat again, "I am," (inhale) pause, "enough" (exhale), pause, "I am," and continue repeating. You can use any other sentence that you want. Please choose something that absolutely serves you. Maybe it's something you want to install into your belief system. Maybe you like, "I am unique" or "I am my breath" or "I am alive" or "I am divine." The goal is to keep all your racing thoughts focused on this single sentence, on *your* sentence. My favorite one is, "I am enough."

You will notice very quickly how your breath slows down when you conduct your breathing to a slower rhythm. Your heart rate will follow almost instantly, and you become relaxed and drowsy and tired. The task is to think just one single thought, and your brain relaxes immediately because it is super easy for your amazing brain to think this one single thought. There is not much effort needed, so the signals are whistled to your glands and organs to reduce the speed, and you feel more and more relaxed. Your mission is to clearly communicate the assignment and hold your thoughts accountable. If your thoughts start to wander around, bring them back to your mantra, gently but unshakably. "I am enough"; that is all you have to think, over and over and over again, in a very slow pace… and fall asleep.

In case you prefer digits, use numbers and count. One-two with an inhale – pause – three-four with an exhale – pause – one-two – pause – three-four, and so on. One-two – pause – three-four-five-six – pause – one-two – pause – three-four-five-six. That is great. If you can, count up to three with your inhale and four to nine with your exhale.

Ideally, you exhale twice as long as you inhale.

*****

That is impossible for Stella. She is very short on breath, but she can take the lead. She counts in the beginning and switches to her mantra, "I am mighty." It works, and she almost falls asleep. Stella is happy, over the moon, and can't wait to crawl under the sheets in her bed at home and sleep, sleep like a baby, like she has not been able to for a very long time. She is in control again.

It's not that she never had sleepless nights again or that she did not have to experience fear or worries again, but she has a tool to govern them. She is no longer overrun by panic attacks and feelings of hopelessness. She can manage her emotions. She can master the fear and handles all the challenges with confidence. And she rests during the day whenever she can afford it, without feeling guilty.

You are in control. You deserve to rest. Recharge. Restore. Regain your confidence. Hush little beautiful soul.

For a quality of life as high as possible, it is very important to control your stress and establish or reestablish a good quality sleep. It is imperative for you to take back control. The information and exercise in this chapter are reliable tools for you, which will help you to regain your balance.

The first step for you is to give yourself permission to be imperfect. Allow yourself to close the gap between expectations and capabilities. Expectations, which might have been created a long time ago and are not serving you anymore, deserve to be reevaluated. Assess your capabilities and circumstances today. Adapt your expectations and your priorities to your current situation. There is no such thing as *absolute* perfection. However, *your* perfection exists. Perfect is what *you* consider perfect.

Please, be gentle with yourself; stretch yourself, but do not burn the candle on both ends.

Just as important as stress-control is sleep – good quality of sleep. You deserve to rest. You need rest and sleep. Again, give yourself permission to take a break, to nap. The wonderful side effect is that you approve this behavior for your loved ones as well. Finding balance between effort and relaxation is essential. You can guide your brain to calm down, and the body will follow. Enjoy sleeping again and supporting your energy-recharge. Your life is going to be much more peaceful after restorative legs of sleep.

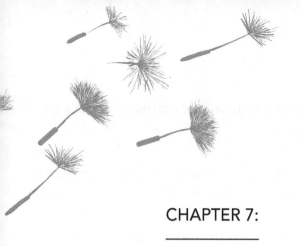

CHAPTER 7:

Love Over Fear

"Imagination is more important than knowledge.
Knowledge is limited.
Imagination encircles the world."
– Albert Einstein

With a good regimen of self-care including high quality sleep, you are more capable of dealing with any situation out of your power center – the solar plexus, just above the navel. That is the place where we usually feel our strongest emotions first. When we have fallen in love, we say, "I have butterflies in my stomach." When we are threatened, we feel angst in the same region. It's also where we get that gut feeling. Sometimes the emotions are so strong that we get sick to our stomach. In a life-threatening situation or after a terminal diagnosis, this is a completely appropriate reaction.

Fear is the feeling we experience when we perceive danger, for instance a disease. It's a very important emotion. We need fear as a warning sign for danger. Without fear, we might jump from a skyscraper. Babies are born with only two fears: the fear of loud noises and the fear of falling. All the other fears, which we experience later in our life, are conditioned reactions. When we feel scared, we develop anxiety and react accordingly. The following actions are freeze, fight, or flight. We all go into freeze state first. Sometimes, it is an unrecognizably short moment before we decide to either flee or fight. This is what happens when the doctor discloses the horrible diagnosis. Do you belong to the majority of people who cannot say anything in the doctor's office – or at least not something meaningful in that specific moment when the merciless fist of the diagnosis hits you? Are you familiar with the questions you ask yourself later at home, in your safe environment: Why didn't I ask the doctor...? Why didn't I question the result? Why didn't I ask about alternative treatment options? Why didn't I...? It's because you couldn't. You were in shock, in a freeze state. Then you went into fight or flight. After a while, you find yourself back to your normal state of brain function, and you enter the cycle of change – denial, bargaining, anger, sadness, acceptance. Your reaction will be vastly influenced by the amount of fear you are experiencing. Depending on how you are conditioned to what you have learned, depending on your previous experiences and your beliefs, you will tackle any challenge or even disease. You can be hindered and blocked by fear, or you can tap into your power and be supported by hope and trust.

You decide.

Fear is without any doubt an adequate emotion to feel in a situation where your life is endangered. The pivotal point is how much power you allow your fear to obtain.

I developed for myself a very simplified model to make it unambiguously clear that *I* have to make a decision. It is a vital decision, and nobody can avoid making this one. The better you understand the interrelation, the better you can make an informed decision, the better you can steer your journey.

Love vs. Fear

If we break all the emotions down to the basic ingredients, we only have two major emotions. Love and fear are the rulers. I am aware that, per scientific definition, love is not an emotion. Nevertheless, love affects us and our behavior significantly.

Imagine the swaying of the two cardinal emotional states as a sine curve. The world demonstrates in many different ways how rhythm works. The seasons of the year, the moon cycle, day and night, high tide and low tide, yin and yang, all have their right to exist, all have their purpose, and all are equally important. We oscillate within our two basic emotions – up and down and up and down or back and forth and back and forth, and so on. If we are in balance, our baseline is the median. We are in the flow with life, and we have approximately the same expansion on each side of the baseline (above and underneath or to the left and to the right). That means the zone of fear is about the same size as the zone of love.

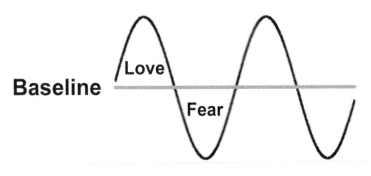

Baseline

Love-Fear Baseline Balanced

Sometimes we live in fear, and sometimes we frolic in the field of love. We can handle both because we have almost equal availability of each of them. If something dramatic happens, a horrible event, a catastrophe, a disaster, devastating news like a diagnosis to be terminally ill or maybe a ruinous thought, the baseline shifts into the segment of love and the area of fear expands radically. Simultaneously, the zone of love diminishes.

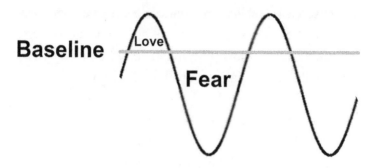

Love-Fear Baseline Shifted

As a result, we dwell in the segment of fear much longer because our fear sector is so much bigger than our love compartment.

What commonly happens is that you continue to gift your loved ones the same amount of love or even more. You continue to invest your love into your job, your hobbies, your pets, your clubs, and charitable organizations regardless of the shriveled availability. What is the result? Whom do you forget? Yes, yourself. Almost unconsciously, you cut off your self-love. Can you imagine how impactful this is, especially if your self-love was already undernourished? On top of that, you have the tendency to stay in the segment of fear because you are familiar with it. It feels safe even though it does not feel good. To feel better again, to be able to enjoy life again and to be happy, you need to change that pattern. What is needed is conscious effort to leave the zone of angst. You need to regain balance. You must re-adjust the baseline to the center. You must return to the flow of life.

You deserve to feel love for yourself. Again, I do not mean selfishness or narcissism. I am talking about self-esteem, self-appreciation. Now, you might think, how can I say that you deserve to value yourself, to love yourself?

I will share with you how I see our life. I learned for myself from my past experiences, including my near-death experiences, that a higher power exists. I call it Source. The home of Source is the Universe. This is my frugal concept of life, the world, and beyond. According to your beliefs, you might want to use another name for it like Divine, God, Allah, Jehovah, Krishna, Father, Mother or others. If you do not believe in a Higher Power, just give it some consideration and be open to my thought-process. I do not want to proselytize you. I simply share with you my view.

Let us imagine that Source gave us the gift of life. We all are gifted with the same gift. We all are alive. We all come from the same parent. Source created us with the same dedication. We all are created with love. Source loves us all like a parent loves all its children. We all have the birthright to be free and happy. Do you truly think all other people are a good outcome, and Source just messed up with you?!

Now, please take action and put the monster angst into its place. Stop feeding your fear with guilt, shame, and hatred. Focus on love.

I invite you to participate in a little exercise with me. Allow your mind to follow me into a kitchen. This short excursion will explain *how* you can control the fear and manage your emotions.

Advice

If you prefer, you can read it out loud and record it so that you can listen to it later with closed eyes and let your mind slip in even further. Or have someone read it to you, if possible.

Either way, enjoy!

Exercise: Lemon

*****

Breathe softly. Inhale and exhale very gentle. With every exhale you feel more and more relaxed. Allow your body to relax. Allow your mind to follow with full focus and try to use all your senses to create a vivid experience.

Now I want you to imagine, to see, to feel that you are in a kitchen. This might be your kitchen or any other kitchen you know very well and you feel good in that kitchen. Maybe several kitchens drift in front of your mind's eye. Pick one and stick with it.

You smell the familiar smell of that kitchen. You know that today, there are fresh lemons in the refrigerator. A wooden board and a little knife sit on the counter top. Now go to the fridge and open the door. You see the light in the fridge and you feel the cold air falling on your skin. You take one of the fresh lemons out of the refrigerator. Now close the door, and you hear the door closing softly, and it shuts tight.

On your walk back to the counter, you are rolling the fresh lemon in between both of your hands. It fills you with joy because you know there is a lot of sour lemon juice with a lot of healthy vitamin C within the lemon. Now you have reached the counter, and you put the fresh lemon on the wooden board. Carefully, you cut the lemon into two halves. You take one of the halves and hold it under your nose. You take a deep breath, and you inhale the fresh smell of the sour lemon. It fills you with joy because you know there is a lot of healthy vitamin C in there.

Now you put the lemon back onto the wooden board and carefully cut a slice off of the lemon. You see a drop of the sour lemon juice running on the wooden board, and you take this slice and hold it under your nose. You take another deep breath now. You inhale deeply, and you smell the fresh smell of this extremely sour and wonderful healthy lemon. And now you are taking a hearty bite in this very sour and fresh slice of the lemon. The intensely sour juice squirts into your mouth. This supremely sour juice squirts on your palate then flows on your tongue, and you notice that your mouth produces saliva, a lot of saliva. And now you feel the urge to swallow. You swallow this pretty sour lemon juice, and it fills you with joy because you have given your body an unexpected extra portion of healthy vitamin C.

Vitamin C helps you to feel energized and makes you feel good.

I want you to take the time to enjoy this wonderful feeling.

Now please take a deep breath. Feel the energy flowing through your body. Take another deep breath and notice how good you feel. Move your fingers. Move your toes. Allow yourself to take another really deep breath. You now feel fully alert, energized, and relaxed all at the same time. You just feel good.

*****

What did you experience? Did you notice that you were producing saliva? Did you have to swallow? You allowed yourself to pretend to bite into that lemon. Yes, you did. Your brain thought of a lemon and the acid. The brain cannot tell the difference between reality and imagination. The imagery itself presupposed you know how a lemon tastes, led you to feel the sourness. As a result of the sourness, your body reacted accordingly by producing saliva because your body wants to protect your teeth against the acid. This all makes sense to our analytical mind, and the cycle is completed. That means it is not a necessity to be guilty of anything or to be threatened; the thought of it is sufficient.

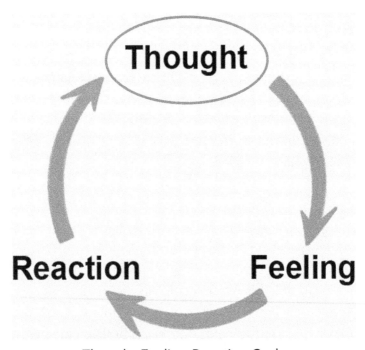

Thought-Feeling-Reaction Cycle

The key is to recognize where that cycle started. It did not start with the sourness in your mouth. It also did not start with salivation. It clearly started with the thought of the lemon. The cycle starts with a thought. *There* we have to intervene when we want to change something. Create the change at the starting point. Change your thoughts. It does not make sense to try to change your feelings first. It does not work out to wait until the fear dissolves. You need to take action. Change how you think. The first cycle is the hardest. When you have completed the new cycle for the first time, your brain can make sense out of the newly created thought > feeling > reaction cycle, and it becomes easier and easier with every single run. This is how you create new neural connections, new neural pathways. This is neuroplasticity put into action. Conquer your excessive angst and walk in blissful love. Keep them in balance.

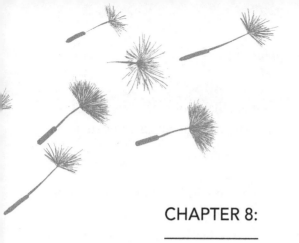

CHAPTER 8:

Killing the Pain With Your Brain

"I am who I am, and I have the need to be."
– Antoine de Saint-Exupéry

Subpoena is derived from the word pain. Pain has its origin in the Latin word poena, which came from the Ancient Greek poiné. In Roman Mythology, Poena was the spirit of punishment and the attendant of punishment to Nemesis, the goddess of divine retribution.

The meaning of pain is penalty or fine, but that meaning is very one-sided. Subpoena has the same genesis, and its synonyms are process, swear out, serve. I think, that it is important to consider this side of the medal. If we see pain as a process, as something that is of service, we can have a completely different approach to managing this summons.

Stella looks at me with her mouth dropped open, literally. She has never ever thought about pain as something that would serve her in any way. She has only felt punished. Stella has felt betrayed by her body. She has felt disadvantaged, deprived, infringed, and violated. After a moment of skeptical thinking, she starts a passionate discussion with me. We both are very engaged and together we develop the general view on pain, the big picture.

The Purpose of Pain

Pain is much more than a punishment and a penalty. Pain is of service. Pain is a symptom of an underlying condition. Pain serves as a warning sign. Pain is the language our body uses in order to communicate with us. Pain is an order. We listen when pain arises. This is the method to catch our attention. Nevertheless, we sometimes make poor decisions after we recognize pain, but at least we register pain. The International Association for the Study of Pain defines pain as "an unpleasant sensory and emotional experience associated with actual or potential tissue damage or described in terms of such damage." Pain is a discomfort.

Childbirth is accompanied by intense pain. It is not a punishment. It clarifies the significance of the event. A new arrival! Pause and acknowledge the paramount importance of that moment - acknowledge the miracle. Pain prompts us to pause.

Pain is the exclamation point, which spirit puts into our essay we call life.

Stella is in complete awe. Stella, as a mother of two, fully understands the deepest meaning of the exclamation point metaphor. She pauses for a moment and rejoices in her epiphany.

Pain is not necessarily your enemy. We are taught that pain is bad. We normally only experience pain as a horrible occurrence which we have to avoid by all means. In other cultures, pain is received as a visitor, a visitor who will leave after a while and not move in forever. You do not have to sign a lease contract with pain; you can just hospitably shelter it for a period of time.

Stella's physical tension melts away visibly, and her emotional tension follows shortly. Her worries and anxieties are diminishing. We continue with our conversation, and Stella understands that our statements hold true for physical pain as well as for emotional pain. She time-travels into the future, to the time when she will not be with her family as a physical being anymore. She sees her loved ones pausing. She sees their lives on hold for a spell. She realizes that a departure is as meaningful as an arrival and that pain has its purpose. It is not about avoiding pain in all circumstances; it is about giving permission to pause. After the stoppage, they will gather their ropes, rebuild their forces, and ascertain how much they have grown. They will grow together, and individually. After the exclamation point, their essays will continue, maybe even more meaningfully. Stella will live on within her family's essay. Her life has meaning. She has meaning. Because she means a lot, those who love her feel horrendous pain about her imminent departure. The meaning is love. It is all about love.

Stella finalizes that she lives her earthly life with meaning until the last second. She makes peace with many different things by understanding the causal connections and realizing to which colossal degree she is the master of her fortunes. She is the main act on her stage. How she approaches pain determines how she perceives it.

That is the control circuit. Here, you control how much joy you allow yourself to feel. Here, you control how you manage the pain; you pilot how peacefully you live and how peacefully you will die later. Until then, live as happily and purposefully and gratefully as possible. Suddenly, Stella grasps that there is no reason to be afraid. Suddenly, she understands. With her mind and her heart, she feels that she is safe. She is the one who navigates.

How to Stop Suffering

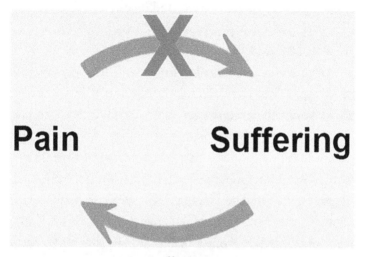

Pain-Suffering Cycle

You cannot always completely avoid pain. What you can do is to not feed the suffering. When you experience pain and give all your attention to it, you can actually increase it because your perception makes you feel that pain more intensely. By giving energy and focus to that misery, you nourish the suffering. Intense suffering leads to intensified pain and so on. Since in some cases, you cannot eliminate the pain, you need to interrupt the cycle between pain and suffering. How much stage presence you allow for the suffering, is your conscious decision. When you interrupt the circuit after the pain, you prohibit the ongoing existence of suffering. The interruption of that cycle, after the pain, leads to starvation of suffering. You can focus on the things again, that you want to strengthen, such as joy, relaxation, peace, and love.

How to Manage Pain

Love is a magical healer. Love can lift heavy weights of struggle. You can decrease the level of pain when you allow yourself to express enough self-love that you can speak your truth. Since pain is of service, we unwittingly accept that pain protects us from doing things we do not want to do. Sometimes, we unconsciously use the presence of pain as avoidance strategy. You have probably heard about the use of headache to not have to have sex. Typically, the woman suffers from a headache, and she really feels the pain and does not have to have sexual intercourse. Sometimes an IBS (Irritable Bowel Syndrome) gets worse just before a family reunion or a large conference the person is supposed to attend. The symptoms are real, no doubt. The only thing is: We could diminish the pain if we spoke our truth and admitted that we do not feel the lust for sex right now or that we do not want to visit the extended family over the holidays or that we do not see the value in attending the conference.

Our body constantly wants to fulfill our wishes, wants to transcribe our thoughts, also the thoughts beyond our conscious awareness. We can dissolve that part of the pain, which is generated by our mind due to avoidance strategy. Become aware of the almost always deeply hidden secondary gain of the symptom and give yourself a great deal of relief. Your mind always works *for* you. You are the director. Direct clearly and truthfully.

Another profound aspect of the level of pain is our expectation. What we have heard, what we might have observed or experienced in our past, has an enormous influence on the perception of pain. If a cancer patient is led to believe that cancer is ruinously painful, how high are the odds that this person will experience unbearable pain? If you as a woman have heard lurid tales about birthing, you probably anticipate a horrible experience of your childbirth. Chances are pretty high that this is what you might have to go through. You do not have to because you decide what you think; you master your thoughts. Thoughts create reality. Your thoughts are going to become your reality. When you do not bite into the terrible stories, when you create your own beautiful experience of the delivery of your baby within your inner mind, chances are very high that you can have a delightful and positive experience of labor.

The Power of Words - The Power of the Mind

The same process goes on in your mind when your MD speaks about your prognosis. How tremendous is the impact of a time prognosis! What happens, when you hear that you have two, maybe three more weeks to live?! In Native American languages, there is not even a term for time. The saying is, "It happens when it happens." In Western culture, we want to hold on to data, to numbers, to facts. Who in the earthly world can predict how long you can live? Who on earth has the right to decide for others how long they might be alive?

Giving a negative prognosis or a time limit after a severe diagnosis was just revealed, is hypnosis. It is installing a new program in the subconscious mind. When a person is in shock, which is the case when a terrifying event happened, the critical factor of the conscious mind is out of order. The information goes directly into the subconscious levels of the mind unhindered. It needs a lot of conscious effort and a good hypnotist to release the disserving program and replace it with favorable suggestions.

On the other hand, the open gateway to the subconscious in the event of shock can be a very beneficial one. If used with discernment and wisdom, it can be lifesaving. From my years as a firefighter I know that every word counts. Every word has a literal meaning. If a victim of an accident hears positive, encouraging words from the first responder, the person has hope and follows the guidance to create a positive outcome within the inner mind. If the opposite happens and the person receives no positive words or information, the mind creates an outcome based on fear and agony. I wish everyone knew about the incredible power of words. I wish everyone knew about the incredible power of the mind.

When pain hits, we have several methods available to cope with it. One method is the use of drugs. Painkillers do actually not kill the pain; they numb the receptors, and due to the numbness, we do not feel the pain. Drugs mask the pain. An unavoidable side effect is the numbness of the mind, too. Be aware that an overly or unneeded use of drugs goes along with the loss of precious power of the mind. Choose wisely and find the best possible combination for you.

Stella proved all her MDs wrong. Stella wanted one year. She outlived her best possible prognosis given to her by exactly 1 year and 63 days, this is 14 months and 2 days, 61 weeks and 1 day, 428 days, 10'272 hours, 616'320 minutes, 36'979'200 seconds. Out of these 14 months and 2 days, she had 11 months and 13 days, which is equal to 95.34% of a year, in really good quality. Her last 80 days were dedicated to her self-determined transition in peace and were carried by love. Who has the right and the capability to decide this crucial question?

You are the only one!

Your marvelous mind is unimaginably powerful. Your mind is capable of creating wonders. It only needs a captain who guides it exactly to the desired destination. When you trust the incredible power of your mind, when you trust yourself and become clear about what you really want, then you can control so much more than you might think. With clarity and willingness to take the lead, you can stop endlessly suffering and diminish or even eliminate unnecessary pain. All too often, we limit ourselves because something seems to be impossible. This is also just a thought; this is just a limiting belief. I encourage you to be bold, to think big. Stop limiting yourself. Discover the power of your mind. Use the power of the words, spoken or intended silently. You own your life; you control it. Live your life with all its boundless possibilities and love.

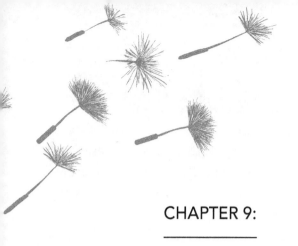

CHAPTER 9:

Forgiveness Is the Golden Ticket

"True love begins when nothing is looked for in return."
– Antoine de Saint-Exupéry

The one year is exactly what Stella needed. I, with my conscious mind to be precise, am not really satisfied in the beginning. My analytical mind calculates with the speed of light the obvious facts and comes to the seemingly logical result that one year is not enough. She is too young, has two children, a good marriage, financial stability, a job she likes, and a cat she adores. Why does she want one more year *only*? I simply have put data, the hard facts, into my equation. I have not considered the soft elements of the calculation. I feel the urge to argue with her about that year. Instead, I manage to just ask her why. Stella looks at me totally astonished and perturbed. "I don't know. I really don't know," she whispers, her head shaking. "It just feels right." I stay true to my own teachings and trust Stella's higher wisdom. With hindsight, I recognize her intuition, although I still struggle with that, although I still miss her dearly, although I still feel the pain of her being in another realm. We agree to use this one year to her best possible interest. Her main goal is to completely understand her life's purpose. She wants to know the why's. She wants to learn her lessons. Words cannot describe how grateful I am to have been allowed to have served and to have been a part of her journey.

All the conscious work has been done already. Stella has lived a deliberate life and since her cancer diagnosis, lived even more intensely. What else can we do? We work in the deeper level(s) of her mind. I use a metaphor to explain our endeavor: The time is right. Stella's most valuable bottle of wine has matured and is ready to be recognized and appreciated. We go into her wine cellar and look for the best, the most precious bottle of wine. Stella discovers it at the bottom shelf in a corner. She grabs the bottle, takes it from the candle-lit, well-tempered secret wine cellar to the table in her cozy sunroom flushed by the warming light of the sun. She carefully cleans the well-aged bottle and looks at it with thoughtfulness. The bottle is beautiful, but the true treasure is embedded within the bottle. To be able to indulge in the special delicacy, we need to open the bottle. We must not shatter the glass because we do not want to lose the wine. We search for the neck of the bottle, gently uncork it, pour the wine in a glass, allow it to breathe. We take the time to explore with all our senses – the sounds of pouring, the color, the smell, the body, and the taste. With every sip, Stella learns to embrace the delightfulness more and more.

To access the deeper meaning and purpose of our life, to fully understand the lessons, to get ready to graduate to the next level, we need to do our home-fun; we need to learn diligently. It takes trust, faith, bravery, and boundless love. Stella's motivation is the love for her family. She knows that she can find peace and graduate gracefully and in dignity when she knows all the important answers. She knows that she can transition and grow in love.

Jacob's incentive was love, too - the love for his wife and daughter, and himself. Love encouraged Marc to fight for their dream. I can give you many, many, many and even more examples from victories of my clients besides my own, thanks to the unthinkable power of love. I want you to have hope! Allow your love to fight and win. Love can do anything. Love can forgive.

Forgiveness is fundamental. Forgiveness is the Golden Ticket to happiness, freedom, and peace. Forgiveness is the one thing that all my clients have had in common:

They all had not mastered it yet. You might think that you are different, and you are absolutely right by thinking it. Everyone is unique. Everyone is special in their own way. I honor and cherish that. However, I have not met a single person yet who has forgiven completely. What we commonly do is to think about the events in our past. We re-examine and analyze and see it from different angles, and when we are really willing to dive deep, we understand many of our life lessons with our mind and our heart. With profound understanding of situations and circumstances, we forgive. Often, we believe the hard work is done, and we sometimes find ourselves astounded when the burden does not get completely lifted. Unfortunately, thorough forgiveness needs more than thinking about the events. Outright forgiveness is much more than a word, much more than a thought. It needs complete devotion to the feeling of absolution. Absolution for oneself, not to be confused with absolution of the perpetrator. All too often, we have the offender on our mind and think or say, "I forgive you," and our focus is on them, on the other person. That is not the core of forgiveness. The heart, the centerpiece of forgiveness is the *I,* the self.

Forgiving Others

It is not about being noble and generous towards the offender. It is also not about downplaying or minimizing the act. It is not to exculpate the culprit of the deed. It is not about sugarcoating anything. Whatever happened to you, whatever hurt you, whoever hurt you, abandoned you, demeaned you, did not treat you well, they have to come to terms with it. You have to find your own inner peace. You have to free yourself from the suffering. The person who hurt you might not remember the event, might not even remember your name or might not be alive anymore. Your forgiving has no influence on the offender, no impact on the delinquent. It is not your responsibility to deliver justice. Your forgiveness has a huge impact for yourself, only for yourself. You are the only person who suffers. You decide how long you continue to carry the burden, the hurt within your heart. You decide when you release yourself from jail. Please take into consideration that when the penalty is paid, when the fine is deducted, the person is permitted to be released from prison. Free yourself! When you have suffered long enough, break the ball and chain, and free yourself.

Forgiveness is not just a term; it is not done by saying the word. Forgiveness is a heartfelt feeling.

Forgiving Yourself

Let us focus on you, please. Bring your emotions along and invite them to passionately partake. Let us have a little conversation and allow me to ask you a question. Have you made mistakes in your life? Your answer is probably, "Yes, of course I have." Sure, we all have made mistakes in our lives. Now I would like to know, how many of your mistakes have you done on purpose?

Give it some thought. With the knowledge you had at that time – with the information, the vision, the experience of life you had at the time when you had to decide – what was your intention? Did you have it on your mind to do something wrong? Did you want to make a mistake? Did you want to hurt someone? Or was it your aim to make it right? Was your intention to do good? What was your goal?

If you think about this, you might realize that you never wanted to fail. You never intended to make a mistake. There's a very high likelihood that not a single one of your mistakes was done on purpose. You simply did not know better. Yes, you probably made mistakes. And yes, they probably hurt you or someone else. This is how we learn. We learn most intensely from mistakes. That is the school of life.

By now, you know forgiveness has nothing to do with playing it down. Forgiveness is the significant decision to free yourself. Forgiveness is the eradicator of guilt and shame. Please symbolically take all your mistakes out of your heart and store them where they belong; store them in your past. It happened. But it happened in your past. Make room in your heart. Forgive yourself. Release the burden, and make room for what you really want to carry within your heart. The heart is the place for love.

Please give all your heart, all your emotions into your self-forgiveness. It is vital for you to restore balance. It is crucial to be able to find peace.

You are enough!

To make sure that you can completely relax and fully understand that you deserve to be forgiven, I invite you to follow along with me to your arrival, to the place, date, and time of your birth. Imagine. Pretend to be that little baby again. Remember, as you were born, were you self-conscious? Did you care that you might be too chubby or too lanky? Did you have any self-doubt? Did you feel any shame or guilt or angst? Did you feel unworthy? Did you feel like a failure? Somewhere down the bumpy road of life, you experienced something, heard something, or felt something that led you to the conclusion that you are not good enough, and you started to repeatedly think those negative judgmental thoughts. You started to feel imperfect. Your thoughts have created your reality.

Jacob honestly believed he was a burden and did not want to live that way any longer. Marc and his wife truly believed they were unworthy of having a baby. Stella honestly believed she could not ask to do things her way because she was not good enough.

When you reactivate your natural cognizance and when you truly trust yourself, then you know – and I mean *really know* – that you are good enough. As you arrived in this lifetime, you did know that you were worthy. With pure self-evidence, you received all the care and protection you needed. You were cleaned, dressed, fed, warmed, and held. Maybe circumstances could have been better. Maybe you would have chosen to live with mom and not be given away for adoption. Or maybe you were born into a large family and had to share mother's and father's attention with a lot of siblings. Maybe your mom was sick and your dad was an alcoholic, or the reverse. Maybe you were born the "wrong" gender. Or anything else did not meet other people's expectations. Maybe you discovered later that something was not 100% satisfying based on someone else's value system. Maybe you had the very best start, the very best parents. I am almost certain that later in life you obtained the impression that you were not a complete success. But for sure, you entered this lifetime with your infinite wisdom of being enough. All your basic needs – air, food, water, sleep, shelter – have been met. That is proven because you are here. You did not have to achieve anything in the beginning of your life to be worthy, to get your needs met. Just because you arrived, just because you are here, just because you are *you*, that is enough. You are enough!

Rediscover your truth. Find back to your very own truth. Rediscover how you entered this lifetime, knowing that you are beautiful, unique, wonderful, perfect, worthy, *enough*. You are enough. That is the truth. Truth heals.

Jacob did, as part of his admirable transformation, incredible forgiveness work. It was not always easy; it was not always fun. However, it was always worth it to shed all the blood, sweat, and tears. He has returned to a life filled with joy, fun, gratitude, and room to evolve. The burden Jacob carries is still about the same, but his attitude is 180 degrees different. The deposition that once was the straw that broke the camel's back is in his past now. Jacob pulled through it with confidence and steadfastness. He stood up for himself, spoke his truth, and was rewarded with respect and fairness. What a triumph! Jacob systematically regained control and happiness in his life. He was able to celebrate a very special anniversary with his beautiful wife. He never stopped loving her, but he had stopped expressing his love to her. She endured all this with him. Love can do anything! Seeing the glow in his eyes, in his striking face – he does not hide it behind a beard anymore – as he talks about her and the surprise he had for their 30th wedding anniversary is priceless. Jacob had chosen the best wife and mother for his magnificent daughter, no doubt. He always wanted to be the very best husband and father in the world. He recovered his energy and courage to be that husband and father, to be himself, to be in balance.

Sometimes, actually in my practices I find this is most often the case, we are not consciously aware of the hurt we carry within our heart. The majority of my clients believe that they have processed the incisive events and have completed their emotional work. What they can catch with the conscious level of the mind, they have done a great deal. I think this is amazing work, and you should unquestionably acknowledge and honor it highly. Our emotions reside in the subconscious level of the mind. To have sustainable, complete forgiveness, you must work in the subconscious level of the mind, which we are capable of doing when we are in hypnosis. Even though hypnosis is a natural state of the mind, I strongly recommend working with a well-trained, trustworthy hypnotist.

Please do not lapse into the misestimation that you have forgiven everything and everyone completely. You probably have not. I know this assumption is daring; anyhow, I bet I am right. We have the tendency to neatly cover our hurt and misinterpret it as solved. I recommend finding a hypnotist you trust and finding out whether there is something left. In case there is, completely dissolve your hurt and make room in your heart for what you deserve to nurture within your chamber of love. Forgiveness is the ultimate gateway to balance, peace, and love.

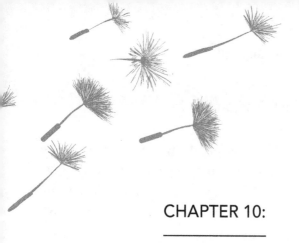

CHAPTER 10:

From Knowledge to Wisdom

"In the middle of difficulty lies opportunity."
– Albert Einstein

Death comes in many shapes and forms. Please make sure that you do not try to die on the inside. You can numb yourself inside. Some become addicted to alcohol or drugs because they think they cannot stand the pain. They want to numb those feelings. The reasons for their feelings do not change by the use of drugs. Their thinking does not either, so the vicious cycle spirals down even more and more. You can stop living happily. You can just vegetate. You can suffer. You can live in agony, but you cannot die inside. Your soul lives on. Infinitely.

How High Is the Price You Pay for Not Actually Living?

What do you miss out on? How many opportunities do you let pass? How much time do you not claim? How many options of treatment do you not demand? How much glory do you miss? How many smiles do you not smile? How many declarations of love do you not hear or say? How much hope do you not feel?

This journey is yours and only yours. You have companions for your ride, some for long periods of time, while others might hop on and off. You are the driver. That is why you need to lead. You can and must ask for advice, request help, demand treatment, beg for support, claim rest, call for relief, but the decision is up to you. If you do not take action, you pay the price. I know it is tough. I also know it is possible and it is worth it! Do not sell your dreams. Create your miracle! Take action. You are not alone. I am here to serve you.

I am fully aware that we have the tendency to remain rigid. It seems to be safer to just keep the same old thing going on. That is, in most cases, not true. It only seems to be safe because it is familiar. Familiar does not necessarily equal good. We are told that change is hard. The more often you hear this, the more you believe it. Just because it is unknown to you does not mean it is bad. Change starts in your head. Be brave and access your inner wisdom.

Knowledge - Science - Wisdom

What I mean by your inner wisdom is to know what is best for you. Do not give up while you still feel a spark hope. As long as you breathe, there is hope.

What you can imagine is what you can create.

Use the power of your marvelous mind.

Create your own unique miracle.

This could be restored health, or it could be a peaceful death. Use the information you have. Question it. Question your prognosis. Gather as much information as you can and organize it. Information organized is knowledge. Based on the definition by Immanuel Kant, accumulated and organized knowledge is science.

What is science? What is the difference between knowledge, science, and wisdom? Two fully committed scientists, my husband and I, having fiery discussions about science, medicine, ancient healing techniques, alternative healing methods, wisdom, and the life after death – can you imagine how blazing this can be?! The word science comes from the Latin word scientia and means knowledge. This is systematically organized information. The data should be measurable, describable, repeatable, and predictable. Here, we come to our disagreement. Medicine is often considered a science. Much data is collected; many parameters are measurable. Some things are explainable. But is it reliably predictable? How do people react to medication? How are the results? What are the potential side-effects? How are the interactions between different pharmaceutical drugs and combinations of them? I often hear from my clients that the prescribed chemotherapy could possibly do this or that or maybe nothing for the patient. Is this considered scientific treatment? I have my doubts.

So, why not add some *not* scientifically proven approaches such as the use of crystals? Even though it is not widely described, I have witnessed that the crystal sugilite does a great job for my cancer clients. I cannot say for sure if and what sugilite does for them, but I can confirm that their tumors seem to not like sugilite. If you consider using this crystal, please use it with caution. Sugilite is very powerful. Start with a small piece, and use it just a couple of minutes per day. Increase the time you hold it in your hand very slowly, add one minute or two per day. This, for me, is part of wisdom.

A very appealing story to me is the story about the two wolves. It explains wonderfully how I think that modern Western medicine and ancient healing methods should be used as a complement to each other, in mutual respect and with active communication.

An Old Cherokee Is Teaching His Grandson about Life:
"A fight is going on inside me," he said to the boy. *"It is a terrible fight, and it is between two wolves. One is evil – he is anger, envy,*

sorrow, regret, greed, arrogance, self-pity, guilt, resentment, inferiority, lies, false pride, superiority, and ego." He continued, "The other is good – he is joy, peace, love, hope, serenity, humility, kindness, benevolence, empathy, generosity, truth, compassion, and faith. The same fight is going on inside you – and inside every other person, too."

The grandson thought about it for a minute and then asked his grandfather, "Which wolf will win?"

You might have heard the story ends like this: The old Cherokee simply replied, "The one you feed."

In the Cherokee world, however, the story ends this way:

The old Cherokee simply replied, "If you feed them right, they both win."

He goes on, "You see, if I only choose to feed the white wolf, the black one will be hiding around every corner waiting for me to become distracted or weak and jump to get the attention he craves. He will always be angry and always fighting the white wolf. But if I acknowledge him, he is happy, and the white wolf is happy, and we all win. For the black wolf has many qualities – tenacity, courage, fearlessness, strong will, and great strategic thinking – that I have need of at times and that the white wolf lacks. But the white wolf has compassion, caring, strength, and the ability to recognize what is in the best interest of all.

You see, son, the white wolf needs the black wolf at his side. To feed only one would starve the other, and they will become uncontrollable. To feed and care for both means they will serve you well and do nothing that is not a part of something greater, something good, something of life. Feed them both, and there will be no more internal struggle for your attention. And when there is no battle inside, you can listen to the voices of deeper knowing that will guide you in choosing what is right in every circumstance. A man or a woman who has peace inside has everything. A man or a woman who is pulled apart by the war inside him or her has nothing. How you choose to interact with the opposing forces within you will determine your life. Starve one or the other, or guide them both."

Cherokee Story

Find the best possible way for you. Work together with your medical professionals. Hire a coach. Seek the help of alternative healing methods. Manage your stress. Disarm your angst. Stop volunteering to suffer. Resolve old anger; finish all unfinished business with others. Stop worrying about other people and their judgment. Finish all unfinished business with yourself. Release guilt and shame. Cry all the tears that should have been shed a long time ago. Stop fearing the unknown. Trust your power. Be unstoppable. Clarify whatever is possible for you to get clear about. Learn from mistakes. Forgive! Speak your truth. Fight for your dreams. Hope. Live. Love. Create balance and peace.

Spirit is that part of us human beings that can guide us in unthinkable ways. Spirit has the best, and only the best, intention for us. Whatever we need to learn and experience, Spirit chooses and guides. We only need to listen. I mean *listen*, not just hear. I assume that when you read this book and are still with me, that you have heard Spirit talking to you. This could have been via voice, images, sensations, or knowing, what we often call intuition. The critical point is that we do not stop at receiving the message, the guidance; we should go the extra mile and do what we are told to do.

April – she is now a very dear client of mine – lives with her husband and son in New York City and came to me through her very best friend. Her very best friend lives in Mumbai, India. She came to me when I was asked, for me out of the blue from a person in Mumbai, if I would train and certify hypnotists. Yes, I can and do. Great. The lady would come and take the class with me. Out of fairness, I mentioned that the same method she would learn from me - the OMNI hypnosis method, which I teach at OMNI Hypnosis Training Center® Pennsylvania - is taught and certified in Mumbai by an OMNI hypnosis instructor, too. She knew this already and wanted to be trained by me. I felt very honored. Humbled, I asked Source for the deeper meaning. The answer was to be patient. That was not satisfying to me at all. But I accepted and practiced patience. I am still practicing… Although by now, we know the answer. We had an amazing class, and all the students were very passionate and talented. I, as a nice side effect of the training, was introduced to April. She had cancer. It had started as breast cancer and had severely metastasized. Her lifetime prognosis was just a few months.

April was convinced by her best friend to work with me. I am supremely grateful and touched by April's words, which I am allowed to share with you here:

> *"This is one of those miracle stories where you don't know how to begin. It is never easy for me to put the words correctly and describe my heart on paper. I ask your forgiveness for all grammar and description mistakes.*
>
> *Hypnosis has never been interesting for me; on the contrary it gave me a "run away from it" type of feeling. As someone who has been meditating for a long time, I could never trust anyone to enter my subconscious. If hypnotists could make the patient to stop smoking in a single session, could he/she also make me an addict of some sort? You got the idea…*
>
> *It has been seven years since my breast cancer diagnosis which later spread into metastases in other organs., Eighteen chemotherapy infusions within 15 months, many other cancer drugs, eight PET Scans, a few CT Scans, a couple of emergency*

visits, multiple hospital stays, and many hospital visits happened. My last two years I spent mostly either in the hospital, in my bed, or thinking what was to come next. This was my life. Regardless of my positive attitude, my determination to continue to live and so much desire to get rid of the cancer against all odds, progress was not easy to achieve. In the same hospital, even in the same department, the doctors could not agree on one treatment, surgery, hormone therapy, and/or more chemotherapy. Everything was put on the table to be discussed until I met Petra Frese. Many times, I heard how many months to live I have left if I did not follow certain protocols. Eventually, I established high blood pressure which peaked out the moment whenever I entered the hospital and it stayed up high.

A wonderful friend of mine was going to visit me and join Petra Frese's Hypnosis Certification Program. We went together to Allentown, PA. During the day, she was attending the class, and I was hanging out by myself, doing work, meditating and other things.

At the end of the first day, she was so happy to meet up with me again. "Petra could help you for your cancer!" It took me a while to accept to try hypnosis with my friend's commitment to stay with me during the entire session. And Petra: Her loving attitude, shiny eyes, excitement, made me go for the hypnosis.

We discovered many things which are not good for me and my health already in the very first session. Petra told me I would no longer need sedatives when going through scans and my blood pressure would no longer spike high when I enter hospitals.

Within 36 hours after my first session with Petra, I had to go to the hospital for a PET scan, which was scheduled ten days before. Having the unexpected hypnosis session was a last-minute change of plans regardless of my scheduled hospital visit. As soon as I entered the hospital, they checked my vitals: My blood pressure was 115/79. My last BP was 159/123. I could not believe my eyes. For the previous PET scan, they had to give me sedatives to enable me to go through the machine.

This time without any sedative, I laid down on the bed of the scanner very comfortably; my eyes were open under the machine. I was in shock! Could hypnosis be so effective in one day? One day only?

I had my routine PET scans every three months due to my young age and aggressiveness of the cancer. Each time it became better. My last scan showed a slowdown of the cancer growth in each location, and half of the cancer activity was gone.

My cancer results were so much better immediately. We, my husband and I, couldn't believe it and actually I never believed that hypnosis could be so amazing in just one day to stop the cancer growth. Who could believe this?

Since then, which is around eight months ago, my BP is always around 110/79, never any higher. Also, I never took any sedatives for any scans again.

A few days before I met Petra, my oncologist and another oncologist could not agree on my treatment. Hormone therapy, extra chemotherapy, ovary removal, a new biopsy on the neck... I was so scared, confused, and tired.

After another two sessions of cleansing through hypnosis with Petra, I had all the courage to give medication a break. I thought at the beginning for only one month of a break; one month led to two, two to three. At the end, we were at seven months. Seven months without medicine and I felt great.

At the end of the seven months period, my PET Scan results were so much better, the liver cancer activity dropped by 50%. The radioactive sugar intake was so faint in the lungs, they could not even measure it. The activity in the neck was smaller, and there were no enlarged lymph nodes anymore. The oncologist said, "I was so afraid of that your cancer would completely cover your entire body." The medical doctors never wanted to listen to me.

"I am feeling better. I am feeling better!" They replied, "That's impossible!"

After seven months of the medicine-break, the doctors completely discarded the idea of hormone therapy, removal of the ovaries, and the biopsy in the neck. They were no longer needed.

Petra helped me to regain my lost confidence, my love to my own self, and to take back control of my life again. Petra is a very straightforward person; her shining eyes, her sincere love is unique. I think trustworthy is the best word to describe her. She became the channel of my prayers to God! Oncologists do not see cancer as a psychosomatic disease. They simply want to get rid of the symptoms but not of the real root cause. Which tree can survive by watering, trimming the leaves, and branches without healing the suffering roots?

Cancer is a spiritual transformation. We are spiritual, mental, emotional beings. How can a solution to be expected by surgery, radiation, and chemotherapy only? It is still such a surprise for me that no oncologist ever asked me what I have been doing. But they state with full confidence how they were expecting my body to be completely covered by cancer within that seven months break of medical treatment.

Petra is not a medical doctor, but with her techniques, she knows clearly how to solve our emotional issues which feed the cancer. I am currently still not cancer free, but I am definitely on my way towards that. The doctors' initial goal was just to keep the cancer at bay and make my life longer with so many hospital visits and medical drugs. I am already a living miracle compared to what they have predicted.

Life is beautiful! We should set aside our conditionings and known and unknown fears to open beautiful doors. I am very proud of myself for trusting my best friend and to be brave enough for having my first hypnosis session with Petra.

If you do not have such a great friend like I do, to trust in and who can hold your hand to go to a hypnotist, then trust yourself. You can heal, cure, and even help others.

How can I thank God making Petra the channel of my prayers? How can I thank Petra? No words are sufficient. There are no words.

Thank you, Petra, for integrating my heart into my daily life. Thank you!

Thank you, Petra, for your unbelievable love! No words are enough to describe my gratitude. Life is awesome, as Petra says.

Thank you, God!"

This was written 11 months after we got in touch for the very first time. April is alive! And that is not all; her cancer regresses! We are continuing our work together.

Thank you, Spirit! Thank you, best friend! Thank you, April! Thank you, Source!

CHAPTER 11

Preparing for the Journey Beyond

"It is only with the heart that one can see rightly;
what is essential is invisible to the eye."

– Antoine de Saint-Exupéry

I vividly remember that last day in January as Stella called. It was a beautiful day, cold, snow white, blue sky, sunshine. I saw her phone number, my breath caught, and I picked up the phone without speaking. "It starts now," Stella speaks immediately with short breath and a shaky voice. Her fear has kicked in again. After a short conversation, she calms down, and we arrange to meet for a session. We both know this will be our last one. I ask, "Are you ready?" A tiny pause, a short breath. "Yes." A clear, confident, soft, unshakable, "Yes." Tears surge into my eyes. I am proud of her, so proud of her. She has done her home-fun.

Stella has used her year wisely. She has traveled, not far, but to places she wanted to visit again. She has attended sports tournaments with her kids, has had candle-lit dinners with her husband, cried, laughed, tested her limits, and had many extremely meaningful conversations with friends, family, her cat, and God. On my question whether she has had sex, she grants me a bright smile.

Sexuality is one of our basic life functions like breathing, eating, metabolizing. Many of my clients think a lot about nutrition. They spend a lot of time, money, and energy on getting healthy food. Which is fantastic! Awesome! Do that! But they rarely consider the enormous significance of sex. Being sexually active is a not to be underestimated factor for our well-being. To make it absolutely clear, I do not suggest to just have sex with everyone and everywhere. I simply say that sexuality is a basic element of being alive and needs to be addressed and deserves our attention. We recognize the importance of healthy food in proper amounts and on a regular basis. Nobody thinks that not eating or not drinking water is a good idea. But to stop having sex is okay?!

When you are in a relationship, it is mostly very challenging for the healthy partner to ask for sex. Usually they are frightened of hurting their sick partner. They are terrified that their weakened spouse could break, so they considerately do not attempt to be intimate. The ill partner may interpret this caring, considerate behavior as withdrawal. Maybe due to a changed body, maybe hair loss, weight gain or weight loss, changed mood, weakness, for a ton of possible reasons, they do not feel attractive anymore and seclude themselves even more. The vicious cycle is in place. Another reason for the healthy partner to not initiate intimacy could be a conscious or subconscious fear of contagion. This fear can occur whether it is a contagious ailment or not. And again, the vicious cycle is on. Maybe the healthy partner needs to talk to your doctor or do more detailed research about this specific situation. Be extremely selective with whom you share your sexuality or if you share it at all, but be aware of the relevance of our basic functions. When you can have a fulfilling sex life with yourself or with your loving partner, please do not miss out on these pleasures. Sexuality and death are very close to each other. They complement each other as complete opposites. Having sex is a clear sign of being alive. Live!

Stella has taken care of the practical things, too. Paperwork also. She has done a lot of planning for her last stretch and has decided on the place where she wants to finish her performance. Stella still needs to decide on *how* she wants to finish her last act. She has organized and communicated everything she could have. No concealing anymore. Open, honest, loving preparation.

My understanding is when everything is learned, when everything is done, when everything is said, when the contract is fulfilled and no unfinished projects are left, the soul can move on and grow. Of course, this is not what we can thoroughly capture with our analytical mind, yet. It is a broad concept of existence, which I interpret in an extremely simplified way.

Before we enter a new lifetime, and we have many lifetimes in stock, we symbolically create and sign a new contract. The contract contains all the lessons we need to learn in our next incarnation. Based on those lessons we agreed to learn, we choose our date of birth, our name, our gender, our parents, family, and circumstances. We choose wisely with the help of guides and Source so that we will be provided with conditions, situations, assets, and affairs which enable us to learn our lessons. The big lessons we recognize are the things we struggle with. The minor lessons or things we have learned in previous lifetimes already, we complete with ease.

Some souls have been on earth many times; they know a lot and have graduated from several stages already. Some other souls are fairly new on earth; they are at the beginning with their learning. I like to compare them as college graduates and kindergarten children. They have very different skills and very different capabilities. This has nothing to do with being better or not; it is simply a question of time, how much time they had available to grow and discover and learn. If they are given the same instruction, let us say to write a four-line poem, what will happen? The kindergarten child is completely overwhelmed and cannot write a single word because it does not know the letters yet. The college student does not have to think long, and the job is done. The college student is able to carry a heavy backpack, symbolically the burdens of life, and needs courage and strength. The kindergarten kid can carry a small and light backpack and also needs to put effort and courage into carrying the backpack and to get through kindergarten. Both work hard, learn a lot, and are exhausted by the end of the day. Neither one of them is lazy. It is not a good idea to exchange their backpacks. The preschooler would not be able to move the heavy one at all, and the sophomore would be bored very soon.

This gives me an understanding why, in some cases, we perceive life as unfair. Some people seemingly have an easy life. One could think that for them, the water streams upwards, and they groan under the weight of life. Others obviously carry a lot, and we might think that they are overburdened and challenged. These assumptions are made based on our human judgment. We do not know, either what contract they have signed or how many lifetimes they had spent on earth before. Maybe this concept is exactly how the Universe works; maybe it is just a construct built on wishful thinking. I am not sure, but I do know for sure that this concept helps me and my clients to cope with life's struggles, tests, and pain.

In the lifetime Stella is about to graduate from, she has learned countless lessons and has passed a myriad of small and big exams. Within the last year, she has gained clarity about the reasons for the things that bothered her the most, the things she had not been able to make sense of before. Now she understands. It does not mean that she needs to like those teasers, but now it makes sense; she understands the meaning of those struggles. That brings her relief! Now she knows with all levels of her being that she is not being punished. She knows that she was able to learn her main lessons and is ready to grow and transition to the next level, into the next realm.

In order to help her make her very last important decision for this life-time, in order to help her decide on *how* she wants to rise to the stars, we dedicate our final session specifically to her transition.

Before we go on entering altered states of mind, I force her to make a promise to me. I obligate her, "Only *half* way. No wiggle room. No negotiations. No arguments. *Half way!*" Amused, she looks at me, gifts me with her beautiful, conversant smile. Stella has no idea what I am talking about but without any hesitation she clearly and assuredly replies, "Yes, I do." We laugh out loud.

To me, this is what counts. This is what a trusting, loving, hardworking client- hypnotist/therapist/coach relationship means to me. Working hard and efficiently together, laughing together, and crying together are, from my point of view, attributes for a constructive, productive, and successful cooperation. I do not feel that crying together with my client would be a sign of weakness. To me, it is a sign of compassion, not pity.

> *"Crying does not indicate that you are weak.*
> *Since birth, it has always been a sign that*
> *you are alive."*
>
> – Charlotte Brontë, Jane Eyre

We both enjoy the moment of happiness and laughter and extend it as long as we can. I guide Stella into the hypnotic state, further and further into the altered states of her mind, and do the same for myself. I connect with her superconscious mind; of course, I have requested approval from her higher states of mind prior to connecting. Spirit allows me to guide her and open the door for her ascension to the stars. We have melted to oneness. We see the same, we hear the same, we feel the same, and suddenly, we know the same. Stella is next to me, with me, and I can see the souls that are awaiting her. I can feel them. I can hear them. Again, my creed got proof. I have taken her to the state of the Plethoric Float™. This state of mind goes beyond human consciousness and allows us to access a higher state of awareness.

Very gently, I bring her back. I help her reconnect with her body and get settled in the here and now. I do not speak a single word. I want her to have the time she needs to process her experience. After a while, Stella turns her head towards me in slow-motion. Her jaw drops, literally.

Still, no word is spoken. She stands up from her reclined chair with no effort, walks over to me, and looks into my eyes intently. "Now, I need you to make me a promise," she says with a resolute voice. I get very nervous. What has happened? I am sure she has experienced exactly the same of what was revealed to me. This was how it always had worked out. What is it that she wants me to promise her?! Stella insists, "I need you to promise something to me!" Okay, reluctantly, I agree. I make a promise. Utterly relieved, Stella slides back onto her chair and exhilaratingly points out, "You need to write a book! You need to tell the world! You need to! People need to know!" Here I am now, keeping my promise. Stella, I honor you. I keep my promise. You continue to live on, in our hearts and in my book.

We have a long, open, intense, and bonding conversation about her experience and the significance and meaning of the message for her and humanity. I am rather self-effacing, and the stage is hers. Stella explicitly explains what she has seen, heard, felt. In depth, she describes the beauty of the trip, the light, the freedom, and the unconditional love she felt. She can name the souls who are waiting for her. She can feel the wonderful loving expectation for her to arrive over there. Everything is prepared and ready for her transition. She will be welcome. Everything is ready for her to grow, to graduate and mature.

Stella confirms the eminent importance of her promise to me. Temptation to stay there is huge. Stella had exactly the same experience I had. I can listen to her and just nod. In the Plethoric Float™ mind state, we can have oneness when we choose to. We can have individuality if we choose to. We can access the infinite wisdom. What is beneficial for us and humanity is what we can take back to earth and implement in the different levels of consciousness of our miraculous mind.

In retrospect of her excursion to the stars, just half way, Stella summarizes her learnings. Inferentially, she states that she has no fear at all anymore. She is now looking forward to her last act. She knows for sure that she is in control. She now does not fear that she would need to suffer endlessly. In case it would become too hard to stand, she would simply leave her body. She wants to know, whether she could practice, what she has just learned. Yes, as long as you return until it is your time to die, you can rehearse as often as you wish. Stella is excited and assured that she is able to conduct not just her life but also her death. We explicitly recap: Only if all lessons are learned, when everything has come to a conclusion, is she allowed to flower out and travel the full journey. If you do not want to become a repeater, if you want to avoid incarnating with the same lesson(s) again, you are well advised to finish the lectures completely and graduate by passing the exam. The final test is oftentimes to learn receiving. The sooner you accept, the sooner you get permission for your last act and to journey beyond. Take a leap of faith and rise to the stars with peace and love.

Stella retrieved her soul out of her physical body two days before the body stopped working. She passed with full love and self-determination peacefully.

During our last session, Stella, for no obvious reason, took off her scarf and handed it to me followed by softly spoken words, "I think it will suit you nicely." Later, her family had to choose a photo of her for her obituary. They chose a beautiful picture of Stella wearing this particular scarf. Her family had no idea where that scarf had moved to. It might be just a picture; it might be just a scarf, but to me they are much, much more.

To live life deliberately, purposefully, and joyfully cannot be taken for granted. It requires conscious effort and tenacity. Please do not waste time. Please do not hesitate. Live your life with purpose and good intention. Make a difference in the world. Learn your lessons, fulfill your contract, and do not forget to enjoy and to be that joy. By the end of this lifetime, I wish for all of us that we can leave this planet self-determinedly with grace and at peace and travel to the other realm with confidence and love. No fear or uncertainty is needed. We are awaited and welcomed. We are loved. For those who remain here a little longer, I can help you find comfort and hope.

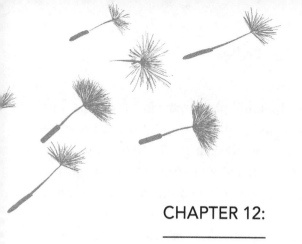

CHAPTER 12:

Flying to the Stars

"Well, I must endure the presence of a few caterpillars if I wish to become acquainted with the butterflies."

– Antoine de Saint-Exupéry

Since I have accepted my calling, I have accompanied many, many souls into the Plethoric Float™ state and beyond. Every single ascension is impressive and unforgettable. Stella represents them all. It is an honor to be granted the opportunity to solemnly hand over a soul to the awaiting escort on the other side. It is absolutely fulfilling to be of service for the souls to grow. These studies led me to completely rethink and reorganize my beliefs about death and dying. I always had severe struggles with the end of life. I felt so extremely sorry for the person who had to leave our beautiful place, our Mother Earth. I was paralyzed by the pain of the bereaved. I did not want to have anything to do with death at all. I did not succeed. I really suffered. I suffered a lot. Now I think it was my fear of the unknown that tortured me. My mind created the worst scenarios. Death as just the ultimate end was one of the best possible options. Just because I did not know about it does not mean that it does not exist. I still feel the pain of each loss. The pain did not lessen, but I do know now that the pain is excruciating only for those who stay back. At the time when we did not have knowledge about the existence of atoms and molecules, they still existed, unimpressed by us not knowing about them. How many treasures exist that we have not gotten introduced to yet? Another example that proves the existence of a bigger outer space is the world of a caterpillar, even though it might not be common knowledge for all caterpillars. The caterpillar probably has no image of the world outside the cocoon. As a result of one of our millions of discussions about my work, my husband, who is remarkably critical and always wants to find scientific proof, surprised me with the following very nice, sweet, loving little story:

Self-Talk of a Caterpillar

Dorothy the caterpillar is crawling across the dirt under the leaves of a nice hydrangea without any blossoms yet. Just the buds provide a hint of how beautiful it will look in gorgeous colors later in the year. It is warm, not hot, and slightly humid, especially in the shadow of the large bright light green leaves of the hydrangea.

A mouse is rushing by, the wind whispering up in the old American walnut trees.

Dorothy is getting forward slowly, trying to avoid the direct sunlight. It feels fantastic to eat from the leaves. A few ladybugs feeding on aphids sit close by. The caterpillar is worried what the future might hold for her.

Is it true that I will not be able to walk around anymore? Is it true that I will be trapped in silk? How does this feel? Is it all over then? The good life?

None of her friends have an answer, but they reinforce her statements. Enjoy life as you do today. Carpe diem!

Who knows what life after this will be? There will be none, most say. It will be over. All the hassle of crawling and feeding – what is it good for anyway? No mating, no kids, no nothing. Still, Dorothy enjoys life with all the colors, sensations, changes of day and night, as well as summer and winter under the surface.

No, it does not go on; we will get trapped in a cocoon. That is our program, and we will die.

Ernesto, another caterpillar, is convinced that life will go on. There will be light. We will soar high. We will travel far. We will find a spouse, and we will have many, many children, and then we will die. This is the best of it all – the next stage. I have heard people calling it butterfly – Monarch, like a royal. So elegant, so divine. That is a better life filled with light and love. Still, there are dangers, but it is worth it. It will be short but better. And if we die, who knows which stage is next?

Does our soul carry on? I do not know. I only know that life after this is better than we can ever imagine, so why do you think that life after being a butterfly is over?

*****

For those who will stay back, I wish you find comfort in my sharing. For those who are about to embark, I wish that you find guidance and confidence.

As mentioned repetitively before, it is crucial to have the right timing. It is impossible to guide a soul over when it is not the right time yet. Source is the sole decision-maker. It is also not possible to naturally hold a soul back when time is up. However, there is, on rare occasions, room for negotiation.

I had a client in her early 60's who was supposed to be ready to transition. Her contract was successfully fulfilled, and it was her time to leave. She suddenly had severe health issues, and it was revealed to me that she would die very soon. In Plethoric Float™ state, I was allowed to negotiate for an addendum on her behalf. Her soul was thrilled and agreed to accept additional tasks, and my client was gifted with more time on earth for this lifetime. She is healthy again and in great shape. This attempt for sure had emanated from a state of ego. Our human judgement is holding us back. At the age of 60, we analytically think that it is too soon because we do not want to live without our loved ones available in physical form. When is it a good age to die? Is there actually an appropriate age?

Our ego is in our way all too often. If we didn't give our egos that much power, we would have so much more joy and happiness. Judgement only happens in the ego-state. Only when we are in ego level, we can compare. Judgement is the result of comparing. When we compare ourselves to others, then we wrongfully conclude that others are better. Others look better, are smarter, have more money, have better careers and are more respected, and so on. We completely disregard that others have other contracts, other lessons to learn. If we took into consideration that we are perfectly made, have the perfect body, the perfect circumstances to learn our lessons and to fulfill the contract, we could be so perfectly in sync and happy with ourselves. Then we would know with all levels of our being that we are enough.

In the moment, we finally are ready to graduate, the soul can ascend even though the body seems to hang on. Those who have to stay back can support the transition tremendously.

A father had completed his tasks. The medical doctors predicted, based on his physical condition, that it would take between two and four more months for him to pass. His son called in tears of deep desperation; he could not see his father suffer any longer. The son's love of his father was bigger than his ego-driven desire to keep him on earth. Less than twelve hours later, the father was peacefully and lovingly released. This shows how miraculous the work in Plethoric Float™ can be. Again, everything only happens with prior approval from Source and the transitioning soul. To surrender a loved one does hurt. A loss hurts. No doubt about this! But the reward of supporting a loved one to suffer less is immeasurable.

How Loved Ones Can Help

The significance of family cannot be emphasized enough. This can determine a curse or blessing for the final act. If time is right, if everything is achieved and death is next, the family has an extreme influence in coloring that process. Spouses, children, and parents are the main factors. When they are willing and able to put love over ego, the process of dying can go really smoothly. Usually it needs the awareness for the importance of that support. I very rarely experience family members who are not able to set the dying person free. Mostly, they are helpless and lost in the overwhelming period. As soon as they are provided guidance, they wholeheartedly serve.

If the person has children and they can be around, they often struggle to find out what to do. They all want to offer the same sort of help. That is not necessary and not the most needed support. Birth order comes into play here. Each sibling has a specific job. No job is more important or valuable than another one. They are equal in reputation for the person who is about to transition. It is wonderfully calming and relaxing when all children find their place in harmony and with no jealousy. The youngest one normally is responsible for the mental joy – the youngest brings the fun. The oldest is the one who should feed, clean the mouth, and lovingly remove the hair from mother or father's face. The middle child is the organizer and communicator with medical professionals. The partner's only job is to hold hands and talk lovingly. It is essential for all to be present. Not necessarily physically, but be present with your heart.

If possible, do not block the position at the foot of the patient's bed.

A client's mother had a stroke. I was consulted and could soothe the family. Mother's time was not right yet; she still had lectures to revue. Contrary to medical opinion, the mother recovered and had many extra months to live. As the second crisis of strokes began, the children again sacrificed themselves for their mother. One daughter turned a deaf ear to all warnings and ran herself into the ground. She ended up in intensive care with very small to zero chances of surviving the generalized infection.

Her body had no capacity for resilience anymore. Instead of allowing her beloved mother to learn the lesson of receiving, she wanted to carry the burden for her. She was almost cited to Source, more than halfway, and would have had to repeat this lifetime's classes. With great efforts, we kept her alive. I really, really hope that she can accept the higher plans. She recovered slowly but steadily. Her father was next. The portal to the stars was open for him for months already. He chose to remain a little longer with his family. The children fulfilled his wish and moved him from Spain to their home country, and he was able to live with his kids. The sisters alternated caring for him in their homes. All spouses and grandchildren and siblings worked together as a team and brought paradise to earth for their father. Now it was his time to go to Heaven, and yet Dad could just stay in paradise. This is another opportunity for my client to learn to lovingly let go or to burn the candle on both ends for herself. I hope that she chooses wisely.

From outside, from eagle's perspective, it is so easy to evaluate. It is very easy to judge. If the lesson is one of your personal main lessons in this lifetime, if you are the focal point in the play, you most likely cannot see the forest for the trees.

The more honestly *all* involved participants give the patient freedom, give their approval to ascent, the easier and smoother the dying process can be. For the person who embarks, it is extremely important that it is an authentic acquittal. Just speaking or thinking the words does not count; it does not do the job. It has to come from the heart with pure love. The tiniest bit of internal conflict will be detected by the patient. All levels below consciousness work intensely. Even though the departing person might not react anymore or is completely unconscious, all other levels of the mind discern everything that is going on or what is not. Please be aware of your language and your emotions. Continue to talk to your loved one; do not stop or hold back because you fear it is pointless. You can speak out loud or simply think what you want to communicate. The soul receives the message. The soul understands everything.

How You Can Continue Communicating

Communication does not stop with departure. Communication will continue open-ended.

The form, the language, changes. Be willing to learn the new language. Pay attention to the signs and hints coming from the other realm. It is very easy to neglect them. Usually those signs are extraordinarily soft. It is super simple to overlook or not hear those signals. The more you trust and ask, the better you will become aware of the assurances from the soul you love and miss so much.

Another way to communicate with the deceased is to communicate in the higher levels of your mind. Hypnosis is a gateway to connect with your late loved one. When you see, hear, or feel with at least one of your own senses, then you believe, then you can heal.

A client's daughter had lost her life in a car accident. My client had sought my services for a different reason. In the intake, she mentioned the loss of her daughter. Me, being a firefighter at that time, immediately knew whom she was talking about. Source, why do you put us in this situation?! Why do we have to start our client-hypnotist-relationship like that?! I struggled! The answer is: to turn it into friendship. With hindsight, the answer is obvious. The mother had coped with her tremendous loss admirably. Years later, I guided her to connect with her beloved daughter's soul to receive the messages she needed to receive to be able to continue to heal. Her daughter explained that she had left her body before it would have been painful. Her daughter did not suffer. She also confirmed, "I am just around the corner." Oh, what a difference. The mother had exactly these ideas in her mind, in her thinking. But now she knows! Now she knows with her heart.

How You Can Help to Allay Grief

After the loss of a loved one, you will not be the same as before. You will not return to the same grade. You will grow. Sooner or later, you need to find back to a new normal. Give yourself permission to feel the pain, but do not hand over the steering wheel to that pain forever.

Take your time and grieve. It is *your* time. That is the exclamation point that Source has put in your life. Pause. There is no rule for right or wrong grieving. There is no prime time or way. The manner of grief is unique like you are. The only universal communality is that you need to allow *all* phases to appear – denial, bargaining, anger, sadness, recovery – and have *all* of them take room and time. Do not skip one. Also face your anger. It is inescapable to let out your anger in order to heal. Sure, you will be marked by scars, but you will overcome this difficult time. Face the shadows. They deserve the same attention as any other pieces because they are essential for balance. It simply does not work to create balance with only one share. We need balance. Balance is healing.

How often do we say something like: That is okay. It is normal. That is life. I knew it for a long time. I had time to say goodbye. He/she is better off now. Or: It was totally unexpected. I do not realize it yet. At least there was no suffering.

That is all true. And that is all only half of the truth. Admit your true feelings. Be honest to yourself. Decide to share your true hurdles with someone. The Universe is sending you some person to listen. Be open to accepting the gesture, the act of friendship. I know this is extremely hard, but please be indulgent with others. You might say that the others do not have the loss, that you have to deal with that void, with that pain. You are absolutely right. However, others have not been trained in dealing with grieving people either. They are probably captured by fear. They do not want to accidentally hurt you even more. They do not know what to say, what to do. You are on their minds and in their hearts, for sure. They usually want to be of help and support for you; they simply do not know *how*. Out of insecurity, they do nothing. They choose to do nothing instead of taking the risk of saying something wrong. Would you be forgiving? Could you take the first step?

To be brave enough and take the first step to ask for help can be vital. It might help someone to come back into happiness and joy of life after a loss. It might even save someone's life. You never know before you do it.

The only thing I do recommend avoiding is saying something like, Time will heal it. It takes time to heal from grief.

Because this is simply not true. Time does not heal. Time puts layer over layer of dust-like covers over the pain, but it does not heal. Actions heal. The best you can do is offer your helping hand, your ears, and your heart to the grieving person. You will know when the person is ready to participate in life again. Gentle pushes, authentic support, and compassionate reinforcement are invaluable.

Anything Is Possible

I was attending a convention in Massachusetts and received a phone call from my husband in Pennsylvania. An internal law for us is that if one is attending a convention or conference, the other only calls in an emergency. I knew right off the bat that something was really urgent.

The partner of a friend of a very good friend of ours had suffered from a life-threatening heart attack. Male, in his 50's, healthy just before the sudden heart attack, in a Southern state. That is all I was provided with. I had met his spouse once. Our mutual friend had called my husband. I was able to connect with the man, Alexander, via those cross ties. His higher mind was awaiting my higher mind. Connection was established immediately. The issue was that he had already traveled farther than halfway. Prospects were anything but good. Since Universe provides what is essential, this happened as I was in great company with other spiritual workers. Instantly, they agreed to help. With united forces, we brought him back. We respected all the rules and made sure that we served for what is best for *him*. We absolutely ensured that we would not work out of ego state. Hours, days, weeks followed filled with ups and downs, hopes and disappointments. Down the road, his condition became so unpromising that his MDs did not see any reason for hope anymore and suggested turning off the life-supporting machines. Even his mother was about to agree. Alexander's spouse and his sister were willing to grab the last straw and listen to my translations. Alexander now wanted to continue with his learning; he wanted to use his second chance. He wanted to live. Against all odds, the two women decided to keep the life support active. Four months later, Alexander was back home living with his partner and allowed to drive the car by himself already. His speed of recovery was phenomenal. Thanks to the love of his partner, thanks to our mutual friend who did not waste a minute, took the leap of faith, and asked for help, and thanks to my husband and my amazing team, Alexander and his girl are happily reunited on planet earth. From the bottom of my heart, I thank my team all over the world! They never questioned me. They never had any doubts. They never complained about my requests for help. They never watched the clock. They never gave less than everything. Thank you, team! You know who you are. They also know I only ask for their powers as long as the situation is imperative.

In contrast to Alexander's situation, I gave advice to a person who cared for a horse, which she had had as her close companion for many years, to release the soul. Her vet still had some ideas for more meds to try. Healthwise, it has been a little less than perfect for a long time already, but medication gave a good deal of stability. Unforeseen, the condition rapidly declined. Emergency visits from the vet, change of treatment, a lot of testing, new medication, and alternative methods did not bring significant relief. One day, my husband and I had breakfast together. All of a sudden, tears filled up my eyes and ran down my cheeks, and I told him out of the blue that I felt the soul leaving the horse's body. I gave him a detailed explanation of that moment. She left her body with extraordinary elegance, performing a pirouette and rising to the stars with grace and weightlessness. I had never seen such elegance and beauty in a transition before. I heard her almost singing voice within me, "I am free now. I am free again. I am done with this heavy body. I am light again." She danced her way up to heaven, happy, free, light. I asked her how she had experienced her life. She laughed and simply said, "It was great! Only my body was too heavy." About two minutes after I had shared the reason for my tears with my husband, my phone rang. The horse's owner – she was in Europe at the time and I in Denver, CO, so we were eight time zones apart – under painful tears informed me about the new situation. She had changed her mind, had trusted my advice, and had the vet release her adored steed instead of prolonging the suffering. Love is stronger than ego. Love can do anything. She continued talking and mentioned that the awful thing was that her steed had fallen backwards. I could explain it to her. Comforted and with bittersweet delight, she confirmed, "Yes, it looked like a pirouette."

To me, life is sacred. I am vehemently against giving up too soon. I advocate fighting, to never give up before the finish line. Whenever it is possible to gain more earthly time, I tenaciously strive for that battle. If everything is learned, if everything is done, then I passionately accompany souls to the next realm, halfway. This is what I do. I do it with unconditional love. It is all about love. The essence is LOVE.

CONCLUSION

"Only a life lived for others is a life worth-while."
– Albert Einstein

Life sometimes treats us nicely. Sometimes, life challenges us to the point that we think it overshoots our capabilities. It is always worth it to bundle forces, accept the test, and move heaven and earth.

With the proper support system in place, eligible methods, suitable attitude, and beliefs you *can* create your miracle. What you think has the potential to become your reality. Imagine! Dream big! Trust your inner power! Never give up before the finish line! Nurture your hope! You can do this!

This book gives you a proven system guideline with practical and easily applicable tools and exercises. When you follow those steps, you have reliable tools to reach your goal. We have touched the most impactful trigger points like treating yourself holistically as the fascinating, unique wholeness you are. Become fully aware of your circumstances and all your options. Take time for your assessment and have an open mind for the wide variety of alternatives. Do not limit yourself; recognize your options, and choose ambitiously. The answer to the question *either* conventional *or* alternative medicine should definitely be *and*. I think and experience frequently that the most successful force is wisely merged science and wisdom. We highlighted not only the importance of speaking your truth and standing up for yourself in order to remove inner conflict for you and to be an easy to care for person to your caregiver; we also emphasized what hypnosis can do for you. Hypnosis is natural yet extremely powerful and a must-have in your treasure chest of tools to create your miracle. We disarmed stress and opened the door for you to rebuild a healthy sleep routine. You received more exercises. Some focus on reestablishing balance between love and fear and why this is so important for your well-being. Pain was our main topic in Chapter 8, and I shared with you how you can break the vicious circle pain-suffering so that you do not have to volunteer for suffering any longer. The master key, the golden ticket, to inner peace is forgiveness. I know how challenging this assignment can be, but I also know how miraculous its results are. You found information, guidance, advice, case studies, and my own experiences and opinions. Please make good use of what might be relevant for you, your loved ones, or the people you care for. Do not yield to despair and grief. Do it your way, but do not give up.

Balance is the desired state of being. In balance, we feel at ease and whole. It is your responsibility and your capability to establish a state of being as close to balance as possible. Including all the different areas of life, facing the shadows, and embracing the joys, will lead you to balance. Oftentimes, especially in times of disaster, heartache, and misery, we need help from outside. Due to distress and pain and worries, we cannot access our full potential, our full power. Chances to succeed are substantially higher when you work with professional aid. Of course, you can do it by yourself. Absolutely, you can follow my guidance and achieve your goals and create balance just by yourself. Brainstorm how much easier it would be if you have assistance. You would receive reinforcement, course corrections, encouragement, and support from an outside view. It would be so much easier to march together, and it would be so much more likely that you arrive at your desired destination when we could master the main connecting stations as a team.

Engage with stress management and minimize the gaps. Stretch yourself for realistic yet high goals. Stress is not your enemy *per se*. You need to control the levels of your stress and build a sustainable system for recharge and recovery. High quality of sleep is essential.

Do not allow the pain, physical or emotional, to drain you in the long run. Establish an unshakable pain management. You are the master of your loop of pain and suffering. Break that continuously ongoing, vicious circle. Maintain self-determination and self-respect. Speak your truth in polite manners and positiveness.

Your miraculous mind has boundless abilities. Trust your mind, and tap into the galactic powers of your mind. Solve all issues at the root; find the causes, and fix them. Restore your natural, innate status. Restore balance. Release all old anger and grudges. Face them bluntly and honestly. That is the prerequisite for liberation. Forgiveness, pure, genuine, heartfelt forgiveness is the golden key to freedom and peace.

When you have given yourself permission to let go of all your judgements, your resentments, and annoyances, you will feel great peace. Make sure that you have nothing left that you regret bitterly. Forgive yourself. You are worth it. Then there is nothing to fear anymore. Life is a journey of learning. Learn and forgive. Live and embark at peace and in LOVE.

In Memory of Stella, our Mommy

After our mother received her life-changing diagnosis of cancer, suddenly everything was different. Our sheltered life turned upside-down from one moment to the next. Our mom, Daddy's wife, the head of the family, was unexpectedly taken away from our well-rehearsed everyday life.

Nothing was the way it was before ever again. Mommy tried to pretend to us children as if everything was fine. But it was not like that anymore! Mommy was terrified, she did not want to leave the house anymore, nor meet people or run any errands or many more tasks she had eagerly carried out before.

One day she told us that she would meet a therapist called Petra. Afterwards, she came home with a smile on her face and raved about how amazing her session was! In the subsequent days and weeks, she underwent a drastic change. She created power again. Slowly but steadily our daily routine came back to our family – with changed roles.

As I found out later, Mom, who never liked to see herself in photos, started to take a selfie every single day. She even put on make-up in the hospital. She gained self-esteem under these brutal circumstances supported by Petra and her counseling.

We had a wonderful time together, being very close and we enjoyed every single moment of it very consciously. We all laughed and we cried, we travelled and went on excursions.

Petra had returned our mother and wife back to us.

Until the very day when Mommy's soul left her body behind.

In the time following her death, it was mainly I and my brother who carried on working with Petra to overcome our grief.

She helped us mourn the tragic loss of our mother and on a positive note she guided me to recognize how tremendously I, my mind and my soul have been growing in this really bad time. Our work together empowered my belief as well as my spirituality. Until then, I had been very skeptical when it came to spiritual beliefs.

The sessions with Petra were very emotional. She guided me in getting through the phases of grief, regaining new power and picking up courage.

Thank you, Petra!

–   Anna with Andy and Dad

REFERENCES

Kübler-Ross, Dr. E., *On Death and Dying*, 1969

Winkler, Dr. A., *Hypnotic Inductions and Prescriptions Handbook*, 1989

Seyle, Hans, "The Stress of Life," 1978

Hooke, Robert, 1635-1703, United Kingdom

FURTHER READING

Hypnosis and Hypnotherapy: Basic to Advanced Techniques for the Professional by Calvin D. Banyan and Gerald F. Kein

Hypnotherapy by Dave Elman

The Hypnosis Treatment Option by Scott D. Lewis

Answer Cancer: Answers for Living: The Healing of a Nation by Stephen C. Parkhill

On Life After Death by Elisabeth Kübler-Ross

My Stroke of Insight by Jill Bolte Taylor

Circle of Life: Traditional Teachings of Native American Elders by James David Audlin (Distant Eagle)

Healing Secrets of the Native Americans: Herbs, Remedies, and Practices that Restore the Body, Mind and Spirit by Porter Shimer

LLewellyn's Complete Book of Chakras by Cyndi Dale

Chakra Healing: A Beginner's Guide to Self-Healing Techniques that Balance the Chakras by Margarita Alcantara

The American Indian Secrets of Crystal Healing by Luc Bourgault

Das Große Lexikon der Heilsteine, Düfte und Kräuter by Gerhard Gutzmann

Herbal Remedies: A Quick and Easz Guide to Common Disorders and Their Herbal Treatments by Asa Hershoff and Andrea Rotelli

The Essential Oils Guide by Teressa Hansch

Medical Medium: Life-Changing Foods by Anthony William

ACKNOWLEDGMENTS

My heart goes out with great gratitude and unconditional love to my husband Dirk who not only saved my life but also saved my love. He does not get tired of shaping and holding his diamond in the rough – me – to the light to get it charged and sparkling.

Beams of love and light to our daughter Vanessa who is my reason to get up every day. Thank you for teaching me to be more brave than fearful. She is our living proof that Herculean thoughts lead to heroic outcomes. Love can do anything.

Deep thankfulness and love fill my heart for my parents who taught me, amongst so many other things, that I need to get up just one more time than I fall down, only one single time.

I thank my in-laws from the bottom of my heart for accepting me for who I am. Thank you for seeing through the clouds and shrugging off all prejudices.

Cold nose, warm heart – these are our Old English Sheepdogs. Late Hazel, thank you for all your love and help to keep our daughter alive. Thank you, Carlotta. She worked herself into my heart and shows to me every day what unconditional love can do. Thank you for being with me all the time, for drying my tears, for sharing my laughter, amplifying my passion, motivating me, and keeping me accountable. Carlotta was lying under my feet until two a.m. every single night whilst I was writing.

"Goodie. Goodie. Goodie." – Thanks to our pet parrot Phoebe who teaches me that loudly speaking my truth is safe and also reminds me that trust and love are not to be taken for granted.

With an honest bow, I thank all my students, clients, colleagues, and my friends. Thank you for helping me to learn undeviatingly. I am thankful for all my friends who know so much about me and go with me through thick and thin. Thank you for your patience, support, input, encouragement, and love. Especially during this writing process, Donna, Doug, Jeanne, Joe, Marco, and Mike, you are my vitamin S (support)!

To all my teachers, I send huge waves of gratitude; first and foremost, to Jerry F. Kein, Hansruedi Wipf, Dr. Anthony De Marco, Larry Garrett and Dr. Pamela Winkler who are my mentors and friends. You are my inspiration. I appreciate you all!

Dr. Angela and team, without you this book would not exist. Dr. Angela, you earned my highest respect. Your competent coaching, Cheyenne's loving guidance, Ora's patient advice, Todd's cheering support, and Ramses' open communication lifted me up. I also want to acknowledge the Morgan James Publishing Team: David Hancock, CEO & Founder; my Author Relations Manager, Tiffany Gibson; and special thanks to Jim Howard, Bethany Marshall, and Nickcole Watkins.

From my soul to your soul – Stella, you obligated me to actually follow through and write this book. Your plea enriched my life and makes you live forever in our hearts. I am thankful for you and your family.

Source, thank you for trusting me more than I do. You gave me the insights for this book. You provide me with courage and strength and humility to accept my calling. You allow me to be of service and live the most important thing in life – LOVE.

THANK YOU

Dear Reader!

Thank you very much for your trust in me and for allowing me to share my thoughts and experiences regarding the power of the mind with you. If you are facing an extremely challenging life-situation and are willing to reach for the stars, then please truly consider getting in touch with me. I am here for you.

> *"The only way to discover the limits of the possible is to go beyond them into the impossible."*
> – Arthur C. Clarke

I honestly wish that you find something in my book that inspires you, gives you comfort, hope, and guidance to overcome a difficult situation. Please share your feedback with me and look for other accompanying programs and updates on my website. www.petrafrese.com

It's all about LOVE!

Yours, Petra

ABOUT THE AUTHOR

A female scientist turned spiritual healer to save her daughter's life – and she did –

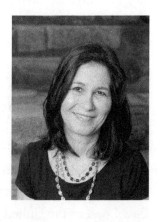

Petra Frese, born and raised in Eastern Germany, dreamed of the West, the Great Plains, and Native American culture as a girl. Studying at the Charité – Universitätsmedizin Berlin among other places to become a scientist, Petra moved to West Germany after the Wall came down. There, she gave birth to her daughter with the life-saving help of her wonderful husband and the medical professionals at the university hospital. Later on, she relocated to picturesque Southern Germany on the Swiss and French border and eventually to Switzerland. She became a pillar of her community as a volunteer firefighter. In addition to that, she also took care of the elderly and supported them while they transitioned to the realm beyond. One of the most decisive events in her life was a sudden and terrible illness that befell her daughter, culminating in a university hospital doctor telling her, "Your daughter will be dying tonight! You better say goodbye!" This experience made her fight harder than ever before in her life – and made her realize along the way she had reinvented a kind of suggestion-based therapy close to hypnosis. Her daughter survived and even learned to speak and walk again, she regained perfect health after the doctors had predicted death and later a life in a wheelchair. This, in turn, led to Petra understanding that she should heal the world by becoming a world-renowned hypnotist and hypnosis instructor with offices in Switzerland and Pennsylvania, USA. She regularly is invited as keynote speaker around the globe. For her lifetime achievements Petra was awarded an honorary doctorate in psychology. She now lives on the East Coast of the United States with her husband, the love of her life, their cold-nosed, warm-hearted dog, and their colorful parrot.

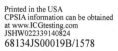

Printed in the USA
CPSIA information can be obtained
at www.ICGtesting.com
JSHW022339140824
68134JS00019B/1578